Handbook of Sports Medicine and Science

Swimming

EDITED BY

Joel M. Stager PhD
and
David A. Tanner PhD

Department of Kinesiology
Indiana University
Bloomington, IN
USA

Second Edition

Blackwell
Science

© 1991 Blackwell Scientific Publications Ltd
© 2005 by Blackwell Science Ltd
a Blackwell Publishing Company
Blackwell Science, Inc., 350 Main Street, Malden, Massachusetts 02148-5020, USA
Blackwell Publishing Ltd, 9600 Garsington Road, Oxford OX4 2DQ, UK
Blackwell Science Asia Pty Ltd, 550 Swanston Street, Carlton, Victoria 3053, Australia

First published 1991
Second edition 2005

Library of Congress Cataloging-in-Publication Data

Swimming / edited by Joel M. Stager and David A. Tanner.—2nd ed.
        p. cm.—(Handbook of sports medicine and science)
   Includes bibliographical references and index.
   ISBN 0-632-05914-1
   1. Swimming–Handbooks, manuals, etc.   I. Stager, Joel McCormick.   II. Tanner, David A.   III. Series.

   RC1220.S8S937 2004
   613.7'16—dc22   2004008705

ISBN 0-632-05914-1

A catalogue record for this title is available from the British Library

Set in 8.75/12pt Stone Serif by TechBooks, New Delhi, India
Printed and bound in India by Replika Press Pvt. Ltd

Commissioning Editor: Andrew Robinson
Production Editor: Nick Morgan
Production Controller: Kate Charman

For further information on Blackwell Publishing, visit our website:
http://www.blackwellpublishing.com

Contents

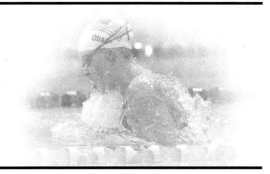

List of Contributors

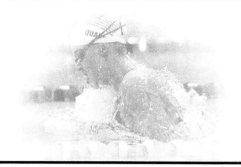

Barry S. Bixler
Principal Engineer, Honeywell Engines and Systems, 3145 W. Tyson Place, Chandler, AZ 85226, USA

Michael A. Coyle PhD
Vice President, Clinical Development, Pharmaceutical Division, VivoMetrics, 100 Overlook Center, Princeton, NJ 08540, USA

David F. Gerrard MD
Associate Professor, Academic Convenor—Sports Medicine, and Associate Dean—Student Affairs, University of Otago, Dunedin School of Medicine, PO Box 913, Dunedin, New Zealand

Wayne M. Goldsmith
Moregold Sports Pty. Ltd, PO Box 112, Charnwood, ACT 2615, Australia

Brendon S. Hale MS
Department of Kinesiology, Indiana University, 1025 E. 7th Street, Bloomington, IN 47405-7109, USA

David B. Pyne PhD
Physiologist, Department of Physiology, Australian Institute of Sport, PO Box 176, Belconnen, ACT 2616, Australia

John S. Raglin PhD
Department of Kinesiology, Indiana University , 1025 E. 7th Street, Bloomington, IN 47405-7109, USA

Joel M. Stager PhD
Department of Kinesiology, Indiana University, 1025 E. 7th Street, Bloomington, IN 47405-7109, USA

David A. Tanner PhD
Department of Kinesiology, Indiana University, 1025 E. 7th Street, Bloomington, IN 47405-7109, USA

Foreword by the IOC

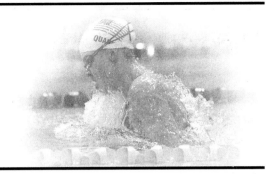

The athlete's health has always been a priority for the International Olympic Committee. I therefore welcome the initiative by the IOC Medical Commission, with Blackwell Publishing, to republish, after 12 years, the *Swimming* handbook.

An Olympic sport since the first Games of the modern era in 1896, swimming has always aroused great interest among both the public and the medical-scientific community.

Through the diversity of its disciplines, and especially because it is practised in an unnatural environment for man, swimming has always been the subject of a great deal of sports-medicine research. This research, both biomechanical and biophysiological, has brought about an improvement in athletes' conditions and training equipment and, consequently, their performances.

I am convinced that this book will be a useful reference tool for sports doctors as well as the medical and paramedical entourage of any athlete. Let us thank the authors for this!

Jacques Rogge
IOC President

Foreword by FINA

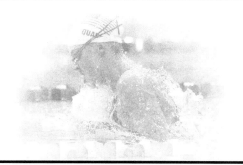

On behalf of the Fédération Internationale de Natation (FINA), it is my pleasure to introduce you to the second edition of *Swimming*, an IOC Handbook of Sports Medicine and Science, which is mainly devoted to the physical, biomechanical, psychological, medical and training problems in competitive swimming. As world governing body for the disciplines of swimming, diving, water polo, synchronised swimming and open water swimming, FINA is obviously interested in the widest possible transmission of knowledge to our athletes, coaches, physicians and officials involved in our sport.

As one of FINA's goals is to disseminate and accelerate the participation of young competitors in our disciplines, it is of relevant importance to detect, correct and prevent the health or injury problems that are inevitably associated with the practice of any physical activity. The engagement in this area led to the creation of a *FINA World Sports Medicine Congress*, held every two years, and to which are invited scientific and clinical experts with an interest in the field of medicine applied to aquatic sports.

We are also proud of counting with the *FINA Sports Medicine Committee* that has the duty of providing medical and sport science expertise and gives recommendations regarding health conditions in the practice of our sports. The professors, doctors and other specialists of this Committee are continuously searching for new ideas and suggestions on how to improve and develop the medical aspects of our aquatic disciplines.

This Handbook, edited by the IOC, is a precious tool to help our members in the prosecution of their activities, as our main goal is to be useful to the aquatic community formed by our 187 Member National Federations. That is why I especially salute the editors and contributors who devoted their time and effort to the elaboration of this publication.

Mustapha Larfaoui
FINA President

Preface

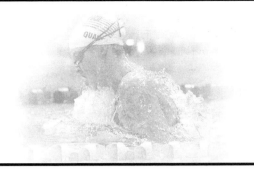

At a recent coaching convention, one of the keynote speakers concluded that nothing particularly innovative has happened within competitive swimming in the last 25 years. The speaker presented evidence that illustrated his point and cited swim goggles, lane lines, interval training, touch pads, pace clocks, and age group swimming as important innovations that acted to transform competitive swimming in the 1950s through the 1970s. It is our hope that while this argument might be seen by some to be valid, the topics presented within this handbook will be cause for this conclusion to be challenged.

The truth is that the world of competitive sports is far from static and is constantly changing. It should be obvious that significant change has resulted from recent advances in science and technology. The history of our sport over the course of the past 100 years of organized competitive swimming is essentially a description of the athletes, their coaches, and their collective accomplishments. In the next decade, however, the history of swimming will be defined by advances in technology, spearheaded by scientific innovators.

In the past year, the world lost two men devoted to innovation and science in swimming. Allen B. Richardson, MD, coauthor of the first edition of this handbook, passed away in September 2003. Then in January 2004 we lost our mentor and friend, James E. (Doc) Counsilman. Both men were committed to improving performance and prolonging the "competitive lives" of swimmers by adapting knowledge from far-ranging fields into the daily routines of swimmers. We, therefore, respectfully dedicate this book to them.

Our association with Doc Counsilman goes back over 35 years and we both admit to have been greatly influenced by his lifelong passion for swimming. Doc often lectured about the "Three C's of Learning: Curiosity, Confusion, and Comprehension." Learning begins with curiosity as to why we do something or how this or that works. Confusion follows when things don't make sense or the rationale behind a practice is found faulty. Comprehension results from repeated observations and the testing of hypotheses. Over the course of time, by asking questions and challenging the *status quo*, advances in knowledge are attained. To paraphrase from Robert Persig, "Scientific truth is not dogma, good for eternity, but a temporal quantitative entity . . . the time spans of scientific truths are an inverse function of the intensity of scientific effort. The more you look, the more you see." Doc Counsilman was most proud of his ability to question, see, and then implement new things that would directly affect how fast swimmers swim.

This is an "up-front" acknowledgment that the *Handbook of Swimming* is not intended for the beginner swimmer. Rather, it is for the serious student of the sport, one with the curiosity and the motivation to delve into the fine details. Some of this material is very complicated, especially the two chapters pertaining to the biomechanics of swimming. Ones first impression might be that the average swim coach does not need to know about symmorphosis or the hydrodynamics of swimming, but the controversy surrounding advances in medicine and the new technologies require that we learn more about fundamental physics and physiology in order to play an active role. It is likely that these chapters will lead to confusion for many of us, but with further study, as Doc suggested, comprehension can be achieved.

We would like to recognize the coauthors of the first edition of this handbook for their fine work: David L. Costill, Ernest W. Maglischo, and the late Allen B. Richardson. We thank the contributing authors of this edition: Barry Bixler, Michael Coyle, Wayne Goldsmith, Brendon Hale, David Gerrard, David Pyne, and Jack Raglin. We commend Nick Morgan of Blackwell Publishing for his patience with us and especially thank Howard G. Knuttgen for coordinating the Handbook of Sports Medicine and Science series.

Joel M. Stager, PhD
David A. Tanner, PhD

Chapter 1
Energy systems

Joel M. Stager and Michael A. Coyle

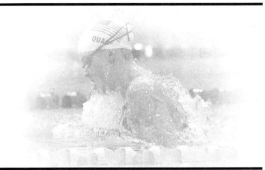

Introduction

Human performance begins at the cellular level, thus the discussion pertaining to the physiology of swim performance must begin there as well. Ultimately, as a swimmer's cells go, so goes the rest of the body. An architect knows that when the bricks of a wall begin to crumble, the building will eventually fall! So too, when the metabolic processes of the cells fail, the swimmer can no longer perform.

The concepts that govern cells and their viability are the same as those that govern the body, its tissues, and organ systems. Tissues are collections of different cell types while organs consist of different tissue types. Organs make up systems and systems make up the body, ultimately constituting a competitive swimmer. How a swimmer adapts to a training regime and the causes of a swimmer's fatigue are determined at the level of the cell; therefore, swim performance is conferred upwards to the complexity level of the entire athlete. The muscle cells are the star performers and the cardiopulmonary, gastrointestinal, renal, and CNS represent the supporting cast.

Regardless of the nature of the response or specific task performed, all physiological work done by a muscle cell requires energy. Although the various cells and cell types of the body are specialized to perform different physiological functions, regardless of the type of work performed, cell metabolism must increase to meet energy needs or work cannot continue. The first point of discussion concerning swim performance and fatigue then is how cells (in particular the muscle cells) supply the energy to do physiological and physical work. Once a basis for understanding is developed, this information can provide a better platform upon which a rational training plan can be built.

Energy for exercise

The ability to increase the mechanical work done by the swimmer is ultimately determined by the ability of the muscle cells to provide the energy to do the work. Whole body metabolic rate can increase more than 40-fold in well-conditioned athletes, with the increased rate of metabolism of the various active tissues (skeletal muscles) being nearly 100 times their metabolic rate at rest. The increase in energy demand is supplied by accelerating the output of several metabolic pathways. The metabolic pathways that provide energy can be separated into those that do not require oxygen, the immediately available phosphogens and glycolysis, and the single metabolic pathway that does, the Krebs or tricarboxylic acid (TCA) cycle (Fig. 1.1). The maximum energy outputs of these three pathways will determine the ultimate performance in swimming events ranging from 50 to 1500 m and beyond.

At rest, a swimmer's oxygen consumption is approximately one third of a liter per minute. The oxygen consumption of mature, elite, well-trained swimmers can exceed $6 \ 1 \cdot min^{-1}$ during near maximal swimming. Estimates of the increase in nonoxidative energy production during swimming are more difficult to make and impossible to measure. Estimates suggest,

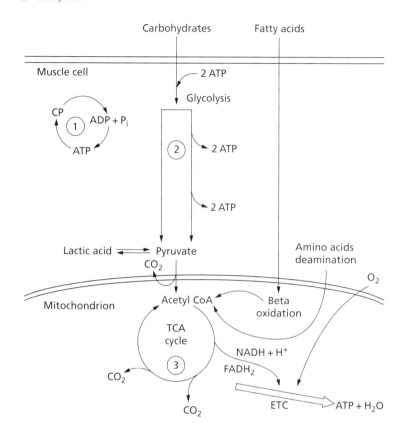

Fig. 1.1 Overview of the three energy systems: (1) Immediate, (2) glycolysis, and (3) aerobic. The immediate ATP–CP system takes place in the cytosol of the cell and produces one ATP for each creatine phosphate (CP). Glycolysis metabolizes glucose in the cytosol, producing a net of 2 ATP and either pyruvate or lactic acid. Pyruvate enters the mitochondria and goes through the TCA cycle. Oxygen (O_2) accepts the hydrogen ions produced by glycolysis and the TCA cycle to result in ATP and water. Fatty acids go through beta oxidation before entering the TCA cycle. Amino acids are deaminated before entering the TCA cycle. The aerobic system produces a net of 36–38 ATP from glucose and 129 from the fatty acid palmitate. ETC: electron transport chain.

however, that a power output that is equal to twice that of the aerobic capacity may be attained by swimmers during "all-out" sprints.

From the perspective of a typical swimming event, two issues are evident. First, although nonoxygen consuming pathways are considered less efficient, they must provide the energy at the beginning of exercise because oxidative (aerobic) metabolism requires several minutes to fully accelerate. There is no way for the cells to anticipate the metabolic power output prior to a muscular contraction. For a short period of time then, at the beginning of a swim bout, there is a deficit between the energy required to do work and the oxidative means to supply it (Fig. 1.2).

Second, energy requirements beyond those which can be provided by aerobic metabolism must come from more than one metabolic pathway. The instantaneous power output that many muscles are capable of performing is greater than that which can be supported by aerobic metabolism. Therefore, at high

exercise intensities multiple pathways are engaged to provide the necessary energy to do work. As is explained later, the greater the nonoxidative energy contribution, the shorter the time this high power output can be sustained.

Source of energy for exercise

Ultimately, the energy to do cellular work is derived from chemical bonds and is contained within the compound adenosine triphosphate (ATP). ATP is produced within each cell from intracellular as well as extracellular substrates. The maximal ATP production of the cell is related to the concentration of reactants, cofactors, and the concentration and characteristics of the various enzymatic pathways.

Under certain circumstances the ability of the cells to produce ATP may be limited by the availability of the

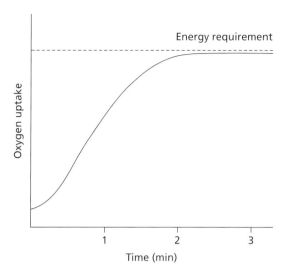

Fig. 1.2 Oxygen uptake as a function of time during intense exercise. During the initial seconds of intense exercise, the difference between the energy required to swim and the energy supplied aerobically is the oxygen deficit.

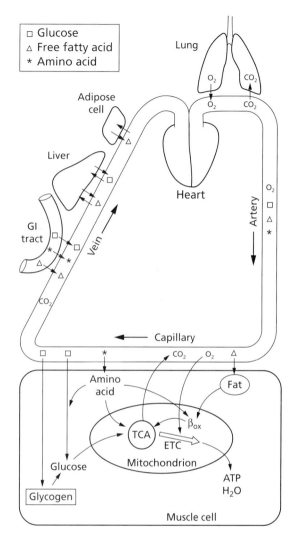

Fig. 1.3 Model of the respiratory system, including the pathways for oxygen (O_2), carbon dioxide (CO_2), and substrates. Carbohydrates, proteins, and fats enter the blood from the gastrointestinal (GI) tract. Glucose and free fatty acids are transported in and out of the liver. The heart pumps blood throughout the body. Oxygen enters the blood and CO_2 leaves the lung. The substrates enter the muscle cell to be metabolized, producing CO_2, water, and ATP. ETC: electron transport chain.

necessary fuel substrates and reactants. At high work intensities, however, most of the fuel for metabolism is from intracellular sources. Delivery of metabolic substrates to the cell is a potential limiting factor only at less intense, more prolonged efforts. It appears, however, that during heavy exercise, the ability of the cardiovascular system to act in this delivery capacity may be the limiting factor in aerobic metabolism. Specifically, oxygen transport, (rather than metabolic substrate transport) appears to limit aerobic metabolism. Rather than the ability of the peripheral tissues to *utilize oxygen*, the evidence suggests that for most athletes it is the ability of the transport system to *provide* O_2 that may limit aerobic metabolism.

The substrates for energy metabolism include carbohydrates, fats, and proteins. Fats and carbohydrates may be stored locally within the muscle cells or elsewhere in specific storage tissues, such as adipose tissues and the liver. Proteins are generally not considered to be "stored" anywhere to any significant extent. They exist as components of the tissues, as circulating entities in the blood, and as compounds absorbed during digestion from the gut, following a meal (Fig. 1.3).

Necessary reactants with all of these substrates during metabolism include oxygen and certain vitamins and minerals that act as coreactants. The important point, however, is that while certain substrates that the body processes into usable energy forms may be stored, ATP itself isn't stored to any great extent. Cells utilize an "on demand" energy system cued by the ratio of substrates to products within the various metabolic pathways. In other words, the ATP necessary for cellular work is generated *when, and only when, there is a demand for it.* The demand is signaled by the presence of the ATP breakdown products adenosine diphosphate (ADP) and adenosine monophosphate (AMP) and by the ratio of ATP to ADP.

Metabolic feed-forward "turbocharger" mechanism

In some ways this "on demand system" is analogous to a turbocharger unit popular on the engines of high-performance automobiles. A "turbo" unit supplies extra air to the engine when demanded by the driver by putting his or her foot to the floor. The compressed air provided by the turbo unit delivers more oxygen to the engine and therefore allows greater fuel combustion for increased power. However, because the turbocharger is spun by the engine's exhaust gases, there must be an increased engine output (more exhaust) before there can be an increased input (more oxygen) from the turbo unit. Some work must be done before increased input can be achieved. Figure 1.4 represents the feed-forward "turbocharger" mechanism of the muscle cell. Aerobic metabolism and glycolysis are fueled by metabolic exhaust in

---

the form of ADP. In order to get the metabolic machinery revved up, some ADP must be created, and the faster ADP is produced, the faster metabolism will attempt to meet the energy needs of the cell.

Metabolic substrates: the phosphogens

Within the cell, prior to the energetic need, there is no way to anticipate the ATP required for subsequent physiological work. There must be a rapidly responding energy production system that reacts quickly to the demand placed upon the cell as a result of work done. The increased energy usage sets into motion increased energy production. Increased cellular exhaust, if you will, signals an increased flux of substrates into the various pathways and energy generation is accelerated to meet the increased need. This initial burst of energy is provided by immediate energy sources within the cells: ATP and creatine phosphate (CP).

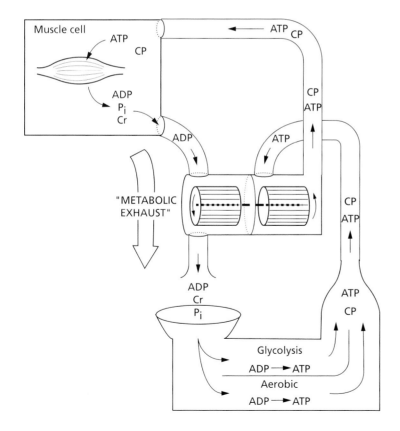

Fig. 1.4 The "turbocharger" model of metabolism. The production of ADP, inorganic phosphate (P_i), and creatine in the muscle cell "primes" the left side of the turbocharger unit, driving the regeneration of ATP and CP via glycolysis and aerobic metabolism.

ATP

So, unlike in a factory where vast stockpiles of raw resources and spare parts are compiled for later use, there is not much room within most cells for maintaining an "energy inventory." This is particularly true for the skeletal muscle cells. Maximal sustained rates of work are not a function of immediately available "stored energy." The limiting factor to extended submaximal performance is the rate at which the raw substrates can be delivered and or converted to usable energy sources.

Thus it is that ATP exists in the body in limited quantities, i.e., there are no vast stockpiles of ATP within the cell or within the body as there is no place to store it. Biochemists estimate that only about 100 g of ATP can be purified from the human body. Roughly half this ATP exists within the skeletal muscles. In contrast, the amount of ATP required to do all of the necessary physiological work done on a daily basis for an average human being is estimated to be *approximately equal to body weight* (about 70 kg)! Interestingly, this is also approximately the amount of additional ATP required to run a marathon or complete a typical two-a-day swim workout.

The breakdown of ATP to ADP and inorganic phosphate (P_i) is enough to provide the initial impulse that signals the acceleration of energy consumption and therefore energy production. But, the immediately available energy sources are barely enough "fuel" to produce a few seconds of intensive effort, although the power output is very high compared to glycolysis and the aerobic pathways. Immediate energy sources can generate power at a rate more than three times that of the TCA cycle and more that twice that of glycolysis.

Creatine phosphate

Creatine phosphate is the other readily available phosphogen and also exists in limited concentrations. Estimates suggest that only about 120 g of CP exist in the body, with most of this found within the muscles ($4 \, g \cdot kg^{-1}$). However, it is important to reiterate that sustained exercise is rarely limited by the immediate availability of ATP or CP, rather, it is the ability to regenerate ATP rapidly which usually sets a limit to prolonged muscular work.

To return to our internal combustion engine model for a moment, everyone can understand that the maximum speed of a car is not a function of how large the gas tank is. It is also true that automotive speed is only partially related to how large the engine displacement is. Semitrucks, for instance, have very large engines but are not necessarily the fastest vehicles on the road. The really high-performance engines depend upon how fast the crankshaft spins (how many revolutions per minute, rpm) and on the engine displacement (piston travel and cylinder volume) to make the car go really fast. Cells that do lots of physiological work have the metabolic machinery that allows recycling of ADP to ATP very rapidly. For a swimmer to swim fast then, it is only partially a function of having a lot of ATP in a large fuel tank. Sprinters, more so than endurance swimmers, rely on the large fuel tank (immediately available phosphogens) to be successful. Endurance swimmers have the ability to convert substrates into energy very quickly. It is this turnover rate, the rate at which ATP can be recycled from ADP or CP, that largely influences mid- to long-distance swim performances.

One important conclusion from this knowledge is that it is virtually worthless to ingest ATP as a means to improve performance. Various supplement products that include ATP in their composition are commercially available. It is unlikely that these supplements are effective given that the ingested ATP would have to be (1) absorbed by the gut, (2) left undigested by stomach acids and enzymes, (3) transported to the metabolically active site via the vascular system, (4) diffused into the metabolically active site, and (5) of enormous quantity. A few slurps of ATP from a small plastic vial represent a very unlikely supplement to a swimmer's premeet diet.

Metabolic substrates: carbohydrates, fats, and proteins

It cannot be said that significant stockpiles of fuel substrates from which energy can be metabolized to form ATP do not exist. Adipose cells, which comprise the fat pads of the body, serve as reservoirs of lipids. Muscle cells have local extracellular fat deposits as well as intracellular lipid reservoirs. Lipids, or rather fatty acids, are available to the cells as particularly efficient fuel substrates. Fat contains roughly twice the energy density per gram of carbohydrates and proteins. It is estimated that average sedentary female may have stored lipids which when processed into energy equivalents might be in excess of 200 000 cal, while the average man may carry the equivalent of 150 000 cal. Given that the average person requires about 2000 cal a day to do the minimum cellular biological work, this stored fat can provide the energy for nearly 100 days. But once again, having lots of fat does not necessarily mean that the capacity to generate energy quickly is particularly great.

In contrast to fats, however, carbohydrates are not stored in peripheral deposits within the body. There are no sugar cubes or subcutaneous sugar crystals that can be felt through the skin. Because carbohydrates represent an important substrate during exercise, they are perceived as limiting to prolonged performances and extended swim practices. Studies suggest that the carbohydrate stores within the active muscle can be easily depleted within a typical swim workout and that the ability to replenish these carbohydrate stores between workouts may be a critical factor in training well.

One of the effects of intensive physical swim training is to adapt the muscle cells to use more fat as a fuel source. This occurs presumably as a means to spare the cell's limited carbohydrate supplies. Because of their importance in fueling exercise, carbohydrate intake is an important parameter to monitor in swimmers participating in multiple workout days and multiple practice days per week. The importance of carbohydrate metabolism should be evident from the extensive interest in the role of lactic acid formation during and following swimming bouts. Lactic acid production comes as a direct result of using carbohydrates as a fuel source to generate energy during an intensive swim effort.

The flip side of elite performance and its understanding is an analysis of the factors that cause fatigue during practice as well as during a competitive swim event. While fatigue is multifactorial, one well-accepted, fundamental cause of fatigue is the inability to maintain the energy requirements of the muscle. A detailed explanation of carbohydrate metabolism via glycolysis is appropriate, as is a closer look at what Brooks *et al.* (1996) refer to as "the mythology of lactic acid."

Three metabolic pathways

There are three pathways for generating energy: the ATP–CP system, glycolysis, and aerobic metabolism. We also know that there are three substrates from which cellular energy can be derived: carbohydrates, fats, and proteins. Finally, we know that each pathway has defined upper limits, or capacities, that are "trainable" to different extents.

ATP–CP: the (nearly) immediately available energy

At the onset of exercise, the first metabolic pathway engaged provides energy derived from the available intracellular ATP and CP within the muscle cell. This pathway involves the phosphogens ATP and CP and a single enzyme, creatine kinase, that catalyzes the reaction between the two. A second pathway, referred to as the myokinase system, generates ATP (and an AMP) from two ADP molecules. It acts to buffer the fall in ATP when energy needs are extreme. Beyond a description of the intermediates and the energetic capacity of the pathway, there isn't much more to be said about the contribution of the immediately available phosphogens. Phosphogen levels increase little with training, essentially in proportion to increases in muscle volume. Estimates of *recovery time* required for this pathway, given a complete exhaustion of the high-energy intermediates, range from nearly instantaneous to 30 s or so.

Current debate surrounds the effectiveness of using creatine and/or phosphate as a means to increase intracellular concentrations prior to exercise. Recent data are inconsistent concerning the ability to increase creatine levels through dietary manipulation. Some reports suggest that increased intake of creatine can enhance power output during short sprint performance through perhaps the 200-m events. The data specifically concerning improvements in swim performance due to creatine supplementation are difficult to interpret as the research designs used in these studies are easy to criticize.

Glycolysis

Glycolysis, the second pathway, metabolizes carbohydrates and involves a series of 12 enzymes and multiple metabolic intermediates (Fig. 1.5). The pathway breaks down glucose as the fuel substrate, requires no oxygen, and ends with the production of ATP and either pyruvate or lactic acid. During prolonged exercise, glycolysis is limited by the availability of carbohydrates as a source of energy. The carbohydrate

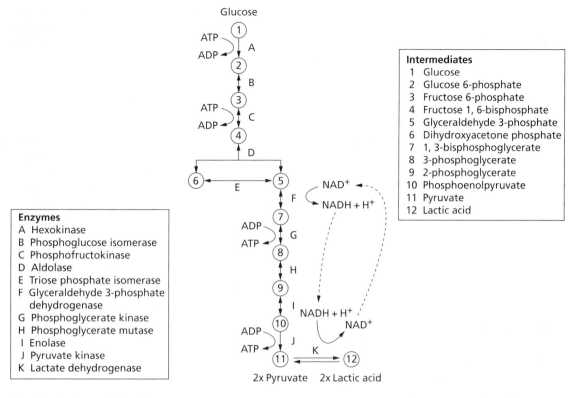

Fig. 1.5 The 12 steps of glycolysis, with associated enzymes.

substrate is either stored within the muscle cell or is transported to the cell through the blood supply. Glucose can be considered a nonoxidative fuel source if the end products are considered to be pyruvate or lactate. Alternatively, glucose can be considered an oxidative fuel source if pyruvate is further funneled through the TCA cycle ending with the products CO_2, H_2O, ATP, and heat.

During intensive exercise and immediately following a meal high in carbohydrate, carbohydrates become the cell's preferred fuel source. In the past, glucose metabolism, or glycolysis, was commonly referred to as *anaerobic metabolism* because oxygen is not directly involved in the process. Today, while still widely used, the term *anaerobic* is considered by some to be a misnomer, or at best, to be misleading. It has led to the belief that glycolysis takes place in the muscles only when there is a lack of oxygen. It is clear, however, that when great amounts of energy are needed quickly, glycolysis plays an important role in providing this energy. Oxygen availability has been determined to have

little to do with the metabolism of glucose or which of the two partial end products, lactate or pyruvate, is produced in greater abundance. It is even known, for instance, that lactic acid is produced at rest, as well as during light exercise, and that the extent to which it accumulates in blood is complex.

Physiological systems tend to be conservative, thus at rest, and several hours after a meal, there is not much glycolysis taking place. Some glycolytic flux, however, is always present to varying amounts in specific tissues and cells. The brain and the red blood cells have little capacity to oxidize fats, thus glycolysis represents the primary pathway for generating energy. The sugars ingested in a meal are used initially as a fuel source, or they replenish storage sites of glucose, or are converted to fat and stored in adipose tissues. In other words, if you have plenty of stored sugars (glycogen) the rest will be metabolized or stored as fat. Most of the energy required by the body at rest relies on the breakdown of fats because fats are abundant and the caloric content of fat makes it an efficient storage form.

In the glycolytic pathway, two net ATP molecules are produced from sugar (commonly a 6-carbon glucose molecule; $C_6H_{12}O_6$) while NAD^+, a vitamin-derived cofactor, is reduced to $NADH + H^+$. NADH is referred to as the "universal hydrogen acceptor" and is important in the electron transport chain (ETC) and oxidative phosphorylation. The final metabolic intermediates of glycolysis are two pyruvate molecules (three carbons each) that are then further metabolized to acetyl-CoA, which funnels through the TCA cycle (within the mitochondria) and is metabolized into six carbon dioxide molecules (one carbon each) and six water molecules (12 hydrogens and six oxygens; $6 \times H_2O$). The NADH equivalents generated in the process are shuttled to the mitochondria for further production of ATP via the ETC (Salway 1995).

If the carbons of the original substrate are followed through glycolysis, a 6-carbon glucose molecule finishes with two 3-carbon molecules of either pyruvate or lactic acid ($C_3H_5O_3$ or $C_3H_6O_3$, respectively). Four ATP molecules are produced in this process but two are required to get the process going. Thus, the net gain in ATP is only two molecules. The big question is: What causes lactic acid to be formed rather than pyruvic acid?

The origin of lactic acid

When glycolytic flux is in excess of mitochondrial uptake (for instance, 15 s after the start of a 100-m freestyle), NADH reduces pyruvate to lactate via fermentation. The enzyme involved is lactate dehydrogenase (LDH) (enzyme K in Fig. 1.5). This reaction is necessary to regenerate the limited supply of NAD^+ needed to maintain a constant carbon flux through glycolysis. In other words, NAD^+ can be considered a limiting factor in glycolysis. When NAD^+ is no longer available, glycolysis will stop halfway. Metabolism of pyruvate, either through the TCA cycle via mitochondrial activity or through its conversion into lactic acid, results in reconversion of NAD^+ from $NADH + H^+$. A high ratio of $NADH + H^+/NAD^+$ will stimulate the conversion of pyruvate to lactate and a low ratio will have the opposite effect.

Glycolysis is able to proceed because lactic acid has been formed from pyruvic acid, thereby regenerating NAD^+ to serve as a coenzyme for glyceraldehyde-3-phosphate dehydrogenase (enzyme F in Fig. 1.5).

Since the pyruvic acid to lactic acid reaction is energetically favorable, fermentation via this route ensures a constant supply of NAD^+ during times when the carbon flux through glycolysis exceeds the mitochondrial capacity to use pyruvate via the TCA cycle. Simply stated, lactic acid will be produced virtually anytime glycolysis takes place regardless of the absence or presence of O_2.

It should be pointed out that if NAD^+ were not regenerated, and all available NAD^+ were reduced to $NADH + H^+$, no ATP could be generated via glycolysis and glycolysis would cease at glyceraldehyde-3-phosphate (molecule 5 in Fig. 1.5). Metabolism would be limited to other fuel sources and power output lowered considerably. Regardless of the cellular environment, in order to keep a carbon flux through glycolysis, NAD^+ *must* be regenerated. It can be concluded, then, that the net formation of lactate or pyruvate depends on the relative glycolytic and mitochondrial flux, and not on the presence or absence of oxygen. The formation of lactate allows the metabolism of carbohydrates to continue, resulting in the rapid production of needed energy to sustain intensive muscular work.

The downside of glycolysis, however, is generally considered to be the accumulation of lactic acid. Once generated, lactic acid at normal pH completely dissociates into a lactate ion ($C_3H_5O_3^-$) and a proton (H^+). As described previously, whenever pyruvate is generated, so too will lactic acid.

Muscular fatigue is a very complex topic. It has been suggested to be mediated, in part, by acidity (a decrease in tissue pH or increased $[H^+]$). The formation of lactic acid, and its subsequent dissociation to lactate, and a positively charged proton (H^+) is a major source of metabolic acidosis during intense exercise. The accumulation of H^+ ions has been associated with a decrement in the ability to produce force in the exercising muscle by interfering with the contractile properties of the muscle, as well as by altering the chemical *milieu* of the cytosolic enzymes. Thus, glycolysis can be inhibited by its own end products, namely the accumulation of hydrogen ions and acidosis.

It may be tempting to conclude that there is no lactate production during swimming if lactate concentration in the blood does not exceed resting levels. At rest and during easy, steady-rate swimming, lactate is produced *and consumed* (i.e., cleared from the blood) at equal rates. As a result, there appears to be no net

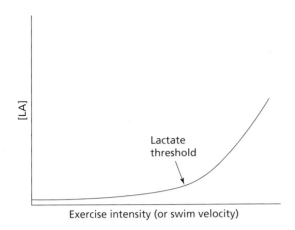

Fig. 1.6 The lactate curve. [LA]: lactic acid concentration.

increase in blood lactate concentration (Donovan & Brooks 1983; Brooks *et al.* 1996). Lactic acid turnover is the ratio between lactic acid production and removal, and infers nothing about the magnitude of the absolute values of either. This lactate turnover (production and consumption) may be several times higher during easy to moderate speed swimming, yet no increase in blood lactate is observed. Intuitively, if lactic acid concentration in the blood increases with increasing swimming velocity, there must be more production than consumption of lactic acid and, hence, lactate accumulates in the blood. At some critical exercise intensity, this begins to be so, as illustrated in Fig. 1.6.

The "anaerobic" threshold

Oxygen consumption ($\dot{V}o_2$) increases linearly with increasing exercise intensity. It reflects TCA cycle metabolism that takes place within the mitochondria. Blood lactate concentration, however, does not change until approximately 65% of $\dot{V}o_{2max}$. This nonlinear relationship results in an inflection point in blood lactic acid at approximately this workload. Historically, this inflection point, *or threshold*, has been referred to as the anaerobic threshold because it was believed that during vigorous exercise, O_2 to the muscle was limited, and the concomitant rise in blood lactate concentration suggested a greater reliance on anaerobic metabolism. More correctly, the lactic acid inflection point, or onset of blood lactic acid (OBLA), represents the balance between the production and removal of lactate from the blood and suggests

nothing about aerobic or anaerobic mitochondrial metabolism *per se*. Importantly, researchers have not been able to show a lack of oxygen in the muscles during exercise intensities above the anaerobic threshold. So what causes OBLA?

The OBLA may be caused by many factors, including any factor that independently influences the production or removal of lactic acid from the blood. Several factors combine to increase lactic acid production and decrease removal during intense exercise. For example, when fast glycolytic fibers (Type IIb) are recruited to contract during intense exercise, they produce lactate regardless of the availability of oxygen (Moritani *et al.* 1984). The autonomic nervous system may influence OBLA as well. Sympathetic stimulation of the pancreas results in the release of glucagon, which, along with epinephrine, results in glycogenolysis in the muscle and liver, respectively. The result is an increase in the availability of glycogen—the fuel for glycolysis. Lastly, adrenergic stimulation and subsequent vasoconstriction of arterioles serve to redirect blood flow during intense exercise so as to maintain adequate cardiac output to exercising muscles, while shunting blood away from the relatively low-metabolic tissues with high resistance to flow (i.e., kidney and liver). The result is reduced blood flow to gluconeogenic tissues (tissues with net uptake of lactate) and diminished capacity for lactate removal from the blood. During very heavy exercise, such as sprint swimming, the blood flow going to the active muscle is 10–20 times more than that which goes to the brain and gluconeogenic tissues. The uptake, or clearance rate, of lactate is thus compromised relative to the rate at which it is being produced.

The fate of lactic acid

The heart and most slow twitch fibers (Type I) have a very high capacity to clear lactate from the blood to the extent that these muscles use lactate as a preferred fuel source. This occurs because there are a number of LDH isozymes (enzyme K in Fig. 1.5) that vary in terms of the direction in which they catalyze the lactate–pyruvate reaction. Those found within the heart and Type I fibers favor the backwards reaction (i.e., lactate to pyruvate), which facilitates the net uptake of lactate from the blood. Indeed, the metabolic fate of most lactate is oxidation via mitochondrial metabolism, resulting in the final products of carbon dioxide and water.

A secondary fate of lactic acid is glucose. Lactate diffuses from the exercising muscle into the capillaries where it is transported, via the blood stream, to the liver (Fig. 1.3). In the presence of oxygen, hepatocytes oxidize lactate to pyruvate that can then be converted to glucose by gluconeogenesis. The glucose can then be exported out of the liver and delivered back to the exercising muscle to serve as a metabolic substrate. This process is known as the Cori cycle and is augmented by another short pathway, the alanine–glucose cycle. In this cycle, alanine, an amino acid, is synthesized in muscle from pyruvate via a transamination reaction. The alanine is released into the blood stream and travels to the liver where it is deaminated to form urea and glucose via gluconeogenesis (Salway 1995).

Thus, lactate should not be viewed as a metabolic waste product, as some authors have stated in the past, but rather as a valuable form of potential energy. Lactate is a source of chemical potential energy that is oxidized during exercise, during recovery, and at rest. It can be converted into glucose and either metabolized or stored as glycogen for later use. This fact is now recognized by several sport nutrition companies. They have recently introduced ergogenic drinks containing lactate as a means to provide a quick energy source for the working Type I muscle and the heart.

Aerobic metabolism

In contrast to the other two pathways, aerobic metabolism can continue to produce energy almost indefinitely. It is much more complex than the non-oxygen using pathways and depends on a robust cardiopulmonary system. The TCA cycle exists within the mitochondria, rather than within the water-soluble cytosol of the cell. Energy production via this pathway requires oxygen as a final proton and electron acceptor plus the ETC (electron transport chain) to phosphorylate ADP (Fig. 1.7). The ETC is located on the inner membranes of the mitochondria. The measurement of oxygen consumption reflects the contribution of this pathway as a source of energy during exercise. The TCA cycle generates NADH and carbon dioxide from the available fuel sources, while the ETC generates ATP from ADP (by shuttling electrons and protons supplied by NADH), and forms energy, water, and heat as final products.

The aerobic pathway begins with acetyl-CoA as the initial substrate. CoA, or more correctly Coenzyme A, is a cofactor and "universal" acetate carrier. The acetate molecule bound to CoA is formed from metabolic substrates (carbohydrate, protein, and fat) as follows: (I) Is derived from the 3-carbon pyruvate molecule when decarboxylated by the enzyme pyruvate dehydrogenase; (II) Is derived from beta oxidation of fatty acids;

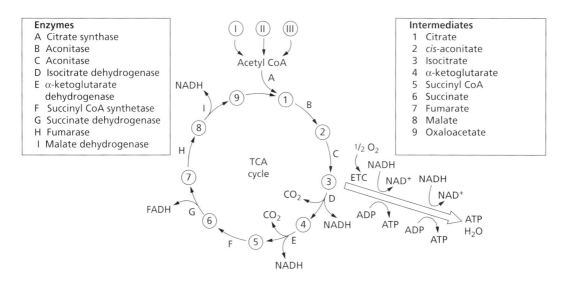

Fig. 1.7 The tricarboxylic acid (TCA) cycle and electron transport chain (ETC). I: Pyruvate; II: acetate via beta oxidation; III: amino acid.

(III) Is a product of the deamination or transamination of amino acids (Fig. 1.7). The function of the TCA cycle can be simplified and described as a pathway that involves ATP production, CO_2 production, and finally, NADH production. The TCA cycle completes the catabolism of glucose, proteins, and fats to the simple compounds CO_2 and water with the assistance of the ETC. The TCA cycle performs the same function for all three primary fuel substrates, by essentially catabolizing acetate to CO_2, ATP, and NADH.

Current understanding is that the substrates needed for mitochondrial metabolism are generally in excess of the capacity of the mitochondria to utilize them. Thus, it does not appear that substrate availability limits maximal aerobic metabolism. The limit seems to be set by the capacity to provide oxygen to the ETC, establishing an upper limit to mitochondrial energy production.

Certainly mitochondrial volume plays a role in this regard. As mitochondrial volume increases, so do the concentration of enzymes involved in the TCA cycle and the ETC cytochromes. Mitochondrial volume seems well matched to capillary density and most other links in the respiratory chain. It appears that the limits to aerobic capacity are shared across the entire system and a good match exists between virtually all variables that could be identified as limiting. A closer look at the factors that potentially limit aerobic metabolism will be made in Chapter 2.

The important concept to reinforce is that the energy required for exercise is fueled through multiple pathways and multiple fuel sources. ATP is the ultimate "exchange unit" in doing work and requires diversified inputs from multiple pathways to sustain the high rate of power output required to perform exercise. As the complexity of the pathway increases (ATP–CP < glycolysis < TCA), the time required to accelerate up to capacity increases as the need for intermediate reactions, optimal concentrations of substrates, and cofactors exists.

In brief, when very intense exercise is required, such as in a 25-m sprint lasting 12 s or less, most of the energy will be supplied in the form of ATP and CP. Because so little ATP and CP exist within the muscle, exercise fueled only by these sources cannot last much longer than this. Glycogenolysis (the breakdown of sugar stored within the muscle) and glycolysis provide most of the energy for longer efforts lasting anywhere from a few seconds to a couple of minutes, by which time aerobic metabolism has ramped up to meet the high-energy demands of the active muscles. Nevertheless, glycolysis continues to supplement aerobic energy sources even during prolonged events.

Relative contributions of aerobic and anaerobic metabolism

There is no easy way of actually measuring the contributions of the three pathways during swimming, and thus, all values provided are estimates at best. Furthermore, a number of additional assumptions must be made in order for us to begins to calculate these contributions.

Each energy system has a different capacity to generate power during swimming. Available estimates suggest that the maximum rate of the ATP–CP system to generate energy is about 36 kcal·min^{-1}. Glycolysis can generate energy at a rate that is roughly half of this or about 16 kcal·min^{-1}. Aerobic metabolism has the ability to generate energy at a rate of only about 10 kcal·min^{-1}. However, the capacities of the three pathways can vary among individuals and within individuals. This means that depending upon genetics and training state, the immediate ATP might supply as much as 50 kcal·min^{-1}. The glycolytic capacity might be nearly 30 kcal·min^{-1} and the aerobic pathway may generate anywhere from 10 to 20 kcal·min^{-1}. The capacity of the immediate and glycolytic energy supplies change by only 10–20% as a result of training but can be affected by differences in muscle mass and fiber type distribution. Aerobic capacity seems to be the most variable and the most "trainable," though the importance of genetics is recognized here as well. Inherited traits and training status might allow for as much as a 50–100% difference among the population in the summated aerobic output capacity of the TCA cycle.

Energy production as a function of event distance

The relative contributions of the three pathways are determined by the intensity of the effort and the

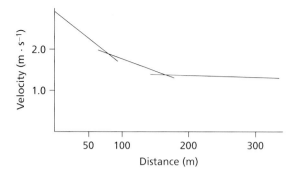

Fig. 1.8 Instantaneous swimming velocity as a function of distance.

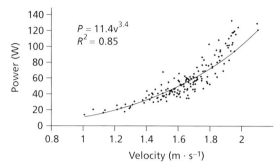

Fig. 1.9 Power as a function of swimming velocity. (Courtesy of Josh White.)

duration of the swim bout. Thus, there is an association between effort intensity, swim velocity, and event duration. From data collected on elite freestyle swimmers, we know that *instantaneous* velocity may be as high as 2.5 m·s⁻¹ in a 50-m race. This maximal velocity drops to 2 m·s⁻¹ when the 100-m races are considered, with instantaneous velocity being somewhat less by the last 10 m of the race. If this is extended out to the 200-m event, the decline in instantaneous velocity continues. The decline in *average* velocity is approximately linear from 50 to 200 m. Thus, the 200-m freestyle is swum at an average velocity that is 20–25% slower than the 100-m freestyle or, about 1.8 m·s⁻¹ (Fig. 1.8). The point to be made here is that metabolic power requirements are related to swim velocity, assuming that changes in mechanical efficiency are not occurring.

In general, the faster a swimmer swims, the greater the energetic requirements. Although the relationship is not linear, as swim events become longer the necessary instantaneous energy requirement drops in proportion to the drop in velocity. One might argue that in fact it is the capacity to generate energy within the cell that drops, resulting in a necessary decline in sustained swim velocity, rather than the other way round.

Velocity vs. power

Because of the nature of the relationship between swim velocity and resultant water resistance (or drag), the power required to swim at any given velocity increases at a rate that is somewhat greater than the square of the velocity (Fig. 1.9). The converse is also

true, the faster the swim velocity, the greater is the increase in the necessary power output. At the shortest competitive distances then, swim velocity is greatest and thus the instantaneous power requirement is also greatest. Power output is so great that short sprints can only be fueled by the immediately available phosphogens.

Because of the energetic capacities of the three metabolic pathways, swim velocity declines in a roughly linear fashion with the increasing event distance, and the power output needed to swim at this velocity decreases at an even faster rate. Therefore, compared to low velocities (or longer distances), at high swim velocities a small decline in speed results in a much greater decline in the energy needed to achieve that speed. The loss of velocity as a swimmer fatigues is buffered by the disproportionate decline in power needed to sustain the reduced swim velocity. That is, "backing off" a little bit at high swim velocities results in a substantial savings from the perspective of energy requirements. This may explain why sprint swimmers rarely, if ever, negative split races.

The opposite perspective, however, is that the faster someone swims the greater will be the necessary increase in the rate of energy production to swim even a little faster. At high swim velocities, the added energetic cost of swimming 0.5 s faster (such as in a 50-m freestyle) might be twice as great as the cost saved by swimming 0.5 s slower. Coaches recognize through experience that the faster the swimmer, the harder it is for that swimmer to go faster still. To a great extent, the basis for this observation lies within the metabolic capacity of the muscle to generate energy and the relationship between swim velocity and drag.

Because of these relationships, the ability to estimate a swimmer's maximal power output allows prediction of that swimmer's maximum swim velocity. To get an idea of the actual power output required to swim at any given velocity consider Fig. 1.9. This figure illustrates the relationship between a swimmer's ability to generate maximum power and their maximum swim velocity (independently measured during a 15-m freestyle sprint). From this it is clear that power output varies greatly among swimmers, as does maximum swim velocity.

Differences are related to the specific characteristics of each swimmer's physique and physiology, although skill may also play a role in this relationship. The better skilled swimmers can generate more velocity requiring less power, in part, because they swim with less drag and use more power to generate effective propulsion. Figure 1.9 also demonstrates how a limited power output can influence maximum velocity. Power output can be constrained by limited muscle mass, muscle fiber recruitment pattern, fiber type and distribution, metabolic pathway enzyme concentration, mitochondrial density and volume, and cardiovascular and pulmonary performance. The importance of these factors changes as a function of event distance, or rather duration, and average swim velocity.

Maximal aerobic capacity

One last topic is necessary to explore before any further conclusions can be drawn concerning energy substrates during swimming. Several lines of research have suggested that the TCA cycle is at maximal capacity ($\dot{V}_{O_{2}max}$) during a 400-m race with a sustained all-out effort. Events shorter than this may not be long enough to allow the TCA cycle to attain maximal output. Events longer than this are swum at lower swim velocities and at $\dot{V}_{O_2}$s that are at or below the necessary threshold velocity. The definition of "threshold" used here is a velocity at which physiological parameters can be held steady and thus any given swim velocity sustained for an extended period of time. If this is so, then it should stand to reason that at the velocity of a 400-m swim, the energy contribution of the TCA cycle is maximal. This does not mean that energy is not being derived from other pathways as well. Because of the low maximal power output of the TCA cycle relative to the immediate and glycolytic pathways, at least some portion of the energy contribution originates from anaerobic glycolysis (perhaps as little as 6% of the total or as much as 60% of the total, depending upon the level of fitness and other physiological traits of the swimmer). For the high-level performer, however, the 400-m event seems to be the distance at which TCA cycle power output is maximized. This distance is used, therefore, when estimates of $\dot{V}_{O_{2}max}$ are obtained from swimmers.

Swimming at any velocity greater than that required for 400-m (i.e., events of shorter duration) requires greater contributions of glycolysis and the ATP–CP system. The point to focus upon is this: the instantaneous power output required at swimming velocities above that achieved in an even paced maximal 400 m is greater than that which can be achieved via aerobic metabolism alone. Because of the time required to fully accelerate this pathway, the 400 m is the shortest event distance that elicits maximal aerobic power output.

As mentioned previously, sprint swimming velocities over shorter distances, such as 10 or 15 m, represent the upper end of power output supported essentially by the available phosphogen sources. Our two points along the metabolic continuum then (the only two which we are fairly sure of) are the all-out 10- or 15-m sprint and the 400-m event.

The Swimgate test of anaerobic power

Figure 1.10 illustrates three typical power output profiles of athletes performing a 30-s all-out effort. This profile is similar to what is seen with running and can be generated during a Wingate Test performed on a cycle ergometer. Hence, the corresponding test for swimming is called a Swimgate Test. The swimmer performs a 30-s all-out effort in the water while attached to an elastic tether. The athlete begins at a distance from the wall that requires maximal force production and attempts to sustain this effort throughout the 30 s. Several interesting characteristics of this curve can be noted. The first is that power output does not peak immediately, but takes 5–7 s. The second is that regardless of motivation or swim effort, power output declines thereafter. Sprinters demonstrate, as might be expected, a greater peak power output. They also display a greater rate of fatigue and finish at a lower

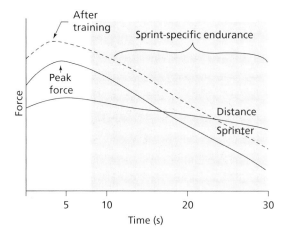

Fig. 1.10 Force production during a 30-s maximal tethered swim for a sprinter and a distance swimmer. The dashed line represents the improvement in force production for the sprint swimmer as a result of a season of training.

percentage of peak power. Distance swimmers cannot generate as much power but their mean power may be similar to sprinters because they can sustain the effort for a longer time. Swim velocities during a swim race do not necessarily demonstrate the "ramping up" profile illustrated in Fig. 1.10, but begin at very high velocities as a result of the velocity gained by the execution of a competitive swim start.

The results of a season of specific power training incorporated into a conventional swim training regime are illustrated by the dashed curve in Fig. 1.10. What appears to occur is an increase in power output throughout the 30-s maximal bout and a more rapid attainment of peak power at the onset of the test. Power output is shown to increase at any given moment suggesting that a greater swim velocity can be sustained, but the decline in the power output, or rate of fatigue, seems to remain about the same. These changes would equate to a swimmer being able to "take it out" faster and sustain a greater velocity throughout a sprint but demonstrate a similar drop in velocity when the front and back halves of the races are compared. This hypothesis would hold for short events such as the 50- and the 100-m events and might only change when discussing events that last beyond 90–120 s. A frequent topic of discussion among coaches is this "sprint specific endurance" and how one goes about improving it. In other words, looking at Fig. 1.10, how can a coach design training so as to reduce the slope of the line in

the shaded portion of the graph, the line that represents fatigue? Surprisingly, there is little evidence to suggest that sprint-specific endurance is improved by a typical swim training program.

Energy systems as a function of swim duration

At the beginning of a short sprint, the energy required to perform the work must necessarily be supported almost exclusively by immediate phosphogen sources. The other two pathways require more time to generate significant power output. Because the combined capacity of the glycolysis and TCA pathways is less than the output of the immediately available phosphogens, maximum swim velocity must necessarily be less at anything beyond this short distance. We will now attempt to estimate the proportional contributions of the three energy pathways as a function of exercise time.

At the start of a race (the first 5 s), or during a short, all-out swim, the metabolic power output above that of rest must come entirely from immediate phosphogen energy sources. There is little contribution from either glycolysis or aerobic metabolism. Using the measures of mechanical power output as a basis, and estimates of efficiency (about 25%), this represents a necessary value of metabolic power output that is on the order of 500 W. This value is lower than that reported for runners and cyclists, perhaps because the arms represent the primary power for swimming while representing a smaller muscle mass than the legs. In addition, swimmers do not work against gravity, rather they work against the resistance of water. They do not support their weight and most of the energy is directed toward power for propulsion. Thus the forces generated by the muscles are substantially less.

Power output is maximal at these initial swim velocities but cannot be sustained for any length of time. As illustrated in Fig. 1.10, both power output and swim velocity begin to decline almost immediately. Energy provided by the immediate sources (ATP and CP) should be considered just that, immediate. The rate of power output is limited only by the kinetics of the reaction, the enzymes involved, and the availability of the phosphogens, i.e., ATP, ADP, AMP, CP, and P_i.

Immediate ATP concentrations last for a few seconds only, with CP acting to buffer the drop in ATP for another 5–8 s. Within 10 s, a secondary source of energy, presumably glycolysis, is needed.

The contribution of glycolysis as an energy source increases quickly and must supplant the contribution of the immediate phosphogen energy sources after the initial 10 s. Glycolysis can be accelerated well before the race begins as neuroendocrine factors initiate responses appropriate for high rates of glycolysis. Physiologic responses appropriate for aerobic metabolism are also invoked (high heart rate and increased ventilation) but the TCA cycle requires more than a minute and a half to reach maximal output capacity.

At 15 s, the swim velocity begins to drop slightly with the immediate sources no longer supplying the predominate contribution to power. But because of the continued high power output requirement, which is greater than the capacity of either the aerobic or anaerobic energy pathways, there must be a very rapid increase in glycolytic activity and a decline in maximal energy generation.

After 20 s or so, the shift toward glycolysis with an increasing contribution from the TCA cycle is nearly complete. It is estimated that the 50-yard or 50-m event is fueled by proportional contributions of approximately 40% ATP–CP, 55% glycolysis, and 5% TCA cycle.

By 30 s or so, the majority of the energy generated to sustain swimming is now from glycolysis. The specific substrate is glucose coming from stored complex carbohydrates located within the skeletal muscle, i.e., muscle glycogen. Rather than being sustained by anaerobic glycolysis, energy is increasingly supplied via aerobic glycolysis.

After 45 s or so, there seems to be another shift in substrate and power production. If the exercise is sustained, a shift toward increased aerobic energy production continues. But, as noted earlier, aerobic metabolism requires nearly 90 s to reach maximal power output. Training helps to move this transition earlier by improving the delivery systems important in providing the substrates for aerobic metabolism. Nevertheless, glycolysis continues to be important, albeit not predominant, through events lasting as long as 10 or 15 min. In fact, aerobic glycolysis continues to be an important pathway providing substrates to the TCA cycle during events lasting several hours or more.

The major difference between short and long events is in how the various products of glycolysis are metabolized. As the relative exercise intensity decreases (as event duration increases), the products of glycolysis are metabolized aerobically through the TCA cycle in equilibrium with the rate at which they are produced.

Events lasting beyond 90 s can be considered dependent upon aerobic metabolism. Glycolysis remains an important early determinant and carbohydrates continue to represent the fuel source. But as swim velocity declines and aerobic metabolism predominates, the training plan needs to focus on developing aerobic capacity to a much greater extent. It is predicted from metabolic traits that success at 400 m and beyond is dependant upon aerobic capacity and that the 200-m events (freestyle in particular) may be a "break point" in this regard. There may be sprinters who can hold on long enough to be successful 200 swimmers and there maybe distance swimmers who can "swim down" and also be successful in the 200 m. These two athletes might be hypothesized to swim very different races. The first might take it out at a high velocity and depend upon a high anaerobic capacity to bring it back while the second athlete might attempt to even split the race and rely on being able to come back when aerobic metabolism supplies the majority of energy. It would further be hypothesized that the optimal training for these athletes should be different. The mistake might be to try and improve the endurance of the sprinter through sustained, short-rest work. It would be expected that while their ability to "come back" might improve, the swimmer's maximal power output might be compromised to the extent that their shorter sprint events may suffer and their overall 200 m time may improve very little. The coach may decide that the swimmer swam a "better" race because of the smaller differential between halves, but there may be little to no improvement in overall time.

Significance of the lactate curve

A considerable amount of information is known about blood lactate concentrations during and following exercise. First, a blood lactic acid profile can be described for each swimmer. This profile represents how blood lactate changes as a function of exercise intensity.

For instance, the type of exercise that will result in high concentrations of lactic acid is short duration intensive swimming or intermittent maximal repeats with long rest intervals (Moritani *et al.* 1984). Conversely, submaximal, steady-rate swimming at a relatively low heart rate and or low percent of $\dot{V}o_{2max}$ does not result in elevated levels of blood lactic acid because of the dynamic balance between lactate production and consumption. This is the type of swimming that should be performed as part of a recovery regime following a competitive event or following a difficult set during a practice. This easy continuous swimming will shorten recovery time. Oddly, the length of the recovery swim needed is inversely proportional to the length of the swim event. Sprinters need to spend more time swimming easily during a recovery swim than do the distance athletes! Recommendations for pace, heart rate, and duration of recovery swims put forth by USA Swimming include the following:

Sprinters	Easy pace (120–130 bpm)	25–30 min
Middle distance	Easy to moderate pace (130–140 bpm)	15–20 min
Distance	Moderate pace (140–150 bpm)	15–20 min

As described previously, there exists a point (OBLA) at which lactate in the blood begins to increase or accumulate. For most untrained individuals, this occurs around 65% of maximum oxygen capacity ($\dot{V}o_{2max}$). However, as the individual becomes trained the OBLA inflection point occurs at a greater percentage of maximal oxygen consumption (Coyle *et al.*1988, 1991; Weltman *et al.* 1992). Highly trained distance swimmers may exhibit OBLA at 90% or more of their $\dot{V}o_{2max}$. This translates to an increased ability to do work at a given workload as well as an increased time to fatigue at a given workload (MacRae *et al.* 1994). This may be a result of an increased ability to clear lactate (lactate consumption), or a reduced reliance upon carbohydrate as a fuel source during exercise, or a combination of both. The interpretation of the lactic acid profile is complex and needs to be considered carefully. A more detailed discussion of the interpretation of blood lactate responses, as well as the balance between aerobic and anaerobic pathway contributions, can be found in a recent publication by Olbrecht (2000).

The role of genetics

We must not overlook the importance of genetics in swim performance. Sprinters, because of their predominant fast twitch glycolytic muscle fiber type, can produce more lactic acid than can most endurance athletes. This is in part because of training programs, but also due in part to genetic factors. Fiber type distribution, largely an inherited trait, plays a role in the balance between lactic acid uptake and lactate production. Sprinters have a lesser capacity to clear lactate and a greater capacity to produce it in part because of their fast twitch fiber types. While lactate uptake appears to be trainable, lactate production rates seem less adaptable. Because there is little evidence linking lactic acid *per se* to muscular fatigue, the significance of high lactic acid levels in the blood is difficult to interpret. Once again, it is the ability to buffer the proton (H^+) produced when lactic acid dissociates to lactate that may limit the continued production of muscular force at high rates of muscular contraction, rather than the existence of lactic acid *per se*.

Lactate and training

OBLA has been shown to represent a good predictor of endurance performance or rather endurance potential. The literature suggests that OBLA is superior to $\dot{V}o_{2max}$ as a predictor of performance and can be used to identify the running or swimming velocity, which is close to race pace (Haberg & Coyle 1983; Fohrenbach *et al.* 1987; Fay et al. 1989; Harrison *et al.* 1992). This suggests that if OBLA can be elevated, training and racing pace can be elevated as well. Improvements in OBLA velocity have also been associated with adaptations in skeletal muscle (Sjodin *et al.* 1982). It can be inferred, then, that kicking drills might be another way to improve lactate clearance following a competitive effort. Any form of exercise that enhances aerobic capacity and/or slow twitch mitochondrial volume might be seen to have this effect. Despite being seen as playing only a small role in propulsion, it may be that the legs, properly conditioned, might play a role as a means of clearing lactate following and perhaps during a swim bout. This might be an additional incentive to include kicking as an integral part of practice for coaches who place little value on it.

Test sets

The purpose of swim test sets such as the T30 or T20, which are evenly paced 20-or 30-min swims, is to estimate the swim velocity that elicits a threshold power output. Threshold refers to a power output that is sustainable indefinitely and represents a break point in the linear increase in physiological parameters, such as OBLA, plotted against swim velocity or exercise intensity. The "threshold" varies as a function of training and exists at exercise intensities somewhere between 60 and 90% of $\dot{V}_{O_{2max}}$. Although little is known about the specific swimming intensity that must be maintained to raise the $\dot{V}_{O_2}$ at which OBLA occurs, Weltman $et\ al.$ (1992) demonstrated that it was better to train slightly above the OBLA threshold rather than at or below the threshold to improve lactate clearance as well as the overall lactate response to exercise. The athlete that wins the 1000 or 1500 m is not necessarily the athlete who has the highest aerobic capacity. All else being equal, it is the swimmer with the highest threshold velocity who has the best chance at winning the race.

Effects of training on the energy pathways

The effect of training, and the purpose of training, particularly during the early stages of the annual training plan, is primarily to increase the capacity of the aerobic pathway. Aerobic sets act to improve the rate at which lactic acid can be cleared. Thus, early season aerobic training forms the foundation for rapid recovery from intensive workouts and multiple events in competition. Increases in aerobic capacity of as much as 50% have been reported. This is somewhat unusual though and is dependent upon the starting point, the type of training, and the capacity of the athlete to adapt. Successful distance athletes have inherently greater aerobic capacities on the order of 50% or more than that of a sprinter. With effective endurance training this capacity can be increased another 20%. Sprinters, in contrast, have a greater glycolytic capacity and thus have

a higher cumulative metabolic power output. The glycolytic capacity is also capable of increasing 20–50% depending upon the inherent characteristics of the athlete and their training regime.

Taking a closer look at the trainability of the immediate energy supply, there is not much to be said. ATP and CP concentrations do not seem to change appreciably with training. Training programs, which incorporate short bursts of very high intensity exercise, do not show significant effects beyond what might be expected with increased muscle mass. The enzyme creatine kinase catalyzing the reaction between ATP and CP is shown to increase in concentration with sprint training. Dietary regimens may act to increase CP levels but intake must be at supraphysiological levels. Concern has been expressed by some trainers about the potential effect this may have upon water balance and kidney function.

It then appears that power output due to glycolysis is dependent upon two factors similar to that of the immediate phosphogen sources: enzyme concentration and reactant availability. With swim training, both variables appear to increase. Greater glycolytic enzyme concentrations will act to increase maximal glycolytic capacity while increased substrate content will increase prolonged exercise endurance.

Finally, endurance training for events lasting beyond 3 or 4 min should be centered upon improving the threshold velocity rather than increasing $\dot{V}_{O_{2max}}$ $per\ se$. The really great endurance performers will have both traits: a high $\dot{V}_{O_{2max}}$ and a high threshold. The route leading toward these outcomes is prolonged, over-distance sets and short rest, sub-threshold sets of relatively high distances per set.

Energy pathways during a swim workout

Short, repetitive bouts of exercise at high intensity can deplete muscle fiber glycogen within 10–15 min. Interval bouts can also rapidly deplete glycogen stores in fast twitch fibers within 20–30 min. Prolonged sustained exercise beyond an hour and a half or so can deplete carbohydrate stores. Exactly when this occurs depends upon many factors such as exercise intensity, previous exercise, dietary intake of carbohydrates, and training state. It is estimated that there are about 300 g of carbohydrate available in the body of a sedentary person with nearly double this amount available in a well-trained, well-fed athlete. When athletes do not consume enough carbohydrates in their diet, swim performance is compromised. Carbohydrates are depleted and declines in performance may be evident as the weekly training plan progresses.

Conclusions

In conclusion, the following points relative to the energy pathways have been addressed. ATP is the ultimate energy source used by the cells to do useful work. ATP cannot be stored to any significant extent, thus most swim performances are determined not by how much ATP exists at the beginning of the race, but by how fast ATP can be regenerated *during the race!* The relative contribution of the energy pathways is a function of the intensity of the exercise bout. Short, maximal efforts lasting less than 10 s are powered by the immediate phosphogen sources: ATP, ADP, and CP.

For events lasting longer than a few seconds, the rate at which ATP can be generated is, in part, a function of the availability of substrates. Depending upon the nature of the training, the specific cellular traits of the swimmer, the swimmer's diet, and the swim event targeted, performance can be enhanced by effecting adaptations that accelerate the rate at which energy, in the form of ATP, can be generated. Alternatively, performance can be improved by keeping substrate levels adequate to meet energy demands and by maintaining the general cellular environment in an optimal status that allows sustained high rates of metabolism.

Lactic acid production is not dependent upon a general lack of oxygen within the body. Tissues such as slow twitch fibers and the heart can consume lactate as a fuel substrate. Perhaps as much as 80% of the lactate produced during exercise is metabolized during the same exercise bout or recovery from it. Lactic acid *per se* has not been shown to be a cause of fatigue and in fact is a convenient, available source of potential energy during exercise. Lactic acid accumulates only when the rate at which it is being produced becomes greater than the rate at which it is consumed.

Aerobic metabolism sustains exercise beyond a minute or so in duration. Improvements in aerobic metabolism may enhance performance in longer events and provide an improved rate of recovery for swimmers specializing in short events.

Chapter 2 will introduce the "delivery" systems that exist in support of the cellular pathways for cellular energy production, and Chapter 3 details the specific skeletal muscle traits within which the mechanisms that represent the means of generating propulsion in swimming exist. In Chapter 8 we will integrate this information and illustrate how these concepts can be applied toward developing a training plan for the competitive swimmer.

Physiological models—A contemporary approach, by David Pyne

The classic model of energy systems evolved over the last 30 or 40 years. However the results of recent scientific investigation combined with practical experience suggest components of this model of fatigue have significant limitations and should be revised. The widely held but somewhat simplistic idea that fatigue develops *only* when the capacity of the cardiovascular systems to provide oxygen to the exercising muscles falls behind the demand, and thereby inducing anaerobic metabolism, is being challenged. Noakes (2000) cites four main limitations of the traditional energy systems model: (i) the heart and not the skeletal muscles would be affected first by anaerobiosis, (ii) no study has definitively established the presence of anaerobiosis and hypoxia in skeletal muscle during maximal exercise, (iii) the model is unable to explain why fatigue ensues during prolonged exercise, at altitude, and in hot conditions, and (iv) cardiorespiratory (maximal oxygen uptake) and metabolic (lactate threshold) measures are only modest predictors of performance. In practice, the experience of swimming coaches and scientists would lend particular support to the latter two limitations (iii, iv) identified by Noakes.

To overcome these limitations Noakes (2000) proposed a new physiological model to explain the complicated phenomena of exercise performance. This revised model consists of the original cardiovascular/anaerobic model and four additional models that regulate short duration, maximal, or prolonged submaximal exercise: (i) the cardiovascular/anaerobic model, (ii) energy supply/energy depletion model, (iii) the muscle recruitment (central fatigue)/muscle power model, (iv) the biomechanical model, and (v) the psychological/motivational model. This revised approach and the concept of integrated modeling is appealing on both theoretical and practical terms. Swimming coaches and athletes understand intuitively that swim performance is multifactorial in nature and the result of a complex overlay of many physical and psychological factors. The evolution of new models of performance (such as that proposed by Noakes) will challenge coaches to devise new and improved ways of preparing swimmers to perform well.

Reference

Brooks, G.A., Fahey, T.D., & White, T.P. (1996) *Exercise Physiology. Human Bioenergetics and Its Applications,* 2nd edn. Mountain View, CA: Mayfield Pub.

Coyle, E.F., Coggan, A.R., Hopper, M.K. & Walters, T.J. (1988) Determinants of endurance in well-trained cyclists. *Journal of Applied Physiology* **64**, 2622–2630.

Coyle, E.F., Feltner, M.E., Kautz, S.A., Hamilton, M.T., Montain, S.J., Baylor, A.M., Abraham, L.D. & Petrek, G.W. (1991) Physiological and biomechanical factors associated with elite endurance cycling performance. *Medicine and Science in Sport and Exercise* **23**, 93–107.

Donovan, C.M. & Brooks, G.A. (1983) Endurance training effects lactate clearance, not lactate production. *American Journal of Physiology. Endocrinology and Metabolism* **7**, E83–E92.

Fay, L., Londeree, B.R., LaFontaine, T.P. & Volek, M.R. (1989) Physiological parameters related to distance running performance in female athletes. *Medicine and Science in Sport and Exercise* **21**, 319–324.

Fohrenbach, R., Mader, A. & Hollman, W. (1987) Determination of endurance capacity and prediction of exercise intensities for training and competition in marathon runners. *International Journal of Sports Medicine* **8**, 11–18.

Haberg, J. & Coyle, E.F. (1983) Physiological determinants of endurance performance as studied in competitive race walkers. *Medicine and Science in Sport and Exercise* **15**, 287–289.

Harrison, J.R., Dawson, B.T., Lawrence, S. & Blansky, B.A. (1992) Non-invasive and invasive determinations of the individual anaerobic threshold in competitive swimmers. *Journal of Swimming Research* **8**, 11–17.

MacRae, H.S.-H., Dennis, S.C., Bosch, A.N. & Noakes, T.D. (1994) Effects of training on lactate production and removal during progressive exercise in humans. *Journal of Applied Physiology* **72**, 1649–1656.

Moritani, T., Tanaka, H., Yoshida, T., Ishi, C, Yoshida, T. & Shindo, M. (1984) Relationship between myoelectric signals and blood lactate during incremental forearm exercise. *American Journal of Physiology* **63**, 122–132.

Noakes, T.D. (2000) Physiological models to understand exercise fatigue and the adaptations that predict or enhance athletic performance. *Scandinavian Journal of Medicine and Science in Sports* **10**, 123–145.

Olbrecht, J. (2000) *The Science of Winning. Planning, Periodizing and Optimizing Swim Training.* Luton, England: Swimshop.

Salway, J.G. (1995) *Metabolism at a Glance.* Oxford: Blackwell Science.

Sjodin, B., Jacobs, I. & Svendenhag, J. (1982) Changes in the onset of blood lactate accumulation (OBLA) and muscle enzymes after training at OBLA. *European Journal of Applied Physiology* **49**, 45–57.

Weltman, A., Seip, R.L., Snead, D., Weltman, J.Y., Haskvitz, E.M., Evans, W.S., Veldhuis, J.D. & Rogol, A.D. (1992) Exercise training at and above the lactate threshold in previously untrained women. *International Journal of Sports Medicine* **13**, 257–263.

Recommended reading

Brooks, G.A. (1986a) Lactate production under fully aerobic conditions: the lactate shuttle during rest and exercise. *Federation Proceedings* **45**, 2924–2929.

Brooks, G.A. (1986b) The lactate shuttle during exercise and recovery. *Medicine and Science in Sports and Exercise* **18**, 360–368.

Brooks, G.A., Brauner, K.E. & Cassens, R.G. (1973) Glycogen synthesis and metabolism of lactic acid after exercise. *American Journal of Physiology* **224**, 1162–1166.

Brooks, G.A., Buterfield, G.E., Wolfe, R.R., Groves, B.M., Mazzeo, R.S., Sutton, J.R., Wolfel, E.E. & Reeves, J.T. (1991) Decreased reliance on lactate during exercise after acclimatization to 4,300 m. *Journal of Applied Physiology* **71**, 333–341.

Burke, L.M. (1996) Nutrition for post exercise recovery. *Australian Journal of Science and Medicine in Sport* **29**, 3–10.

Gaesser, G.A. & Pool, D.C. (1988) Blood lactate during exercise: time course of training adaptations in humans. *International Journal of Sports Medicine* **9**, 284–288.

Hill, A.V. (1914) The oxidative removal of lactic acid. *Journal of Physiology* **58**, **x–xi**.

Hill, A.V., Long, C.N.H. & Lupton, H. (1924) Muscular exercise, lactic acid and the supply and utilization of oxygen. Pt. IV—VI. *Proceedings of the Royal Society B* **97**, 84–138.

Margaria, R., Edwards, H.T. & Dill, D.B. (1933) The possible mechanisms of contracting and paying the oxygen debt and the role of lactic acid in muscular contraction. *American Journal of Physiology* **106**, 689–715.

Sherman, W.M. & Wimer, G.S. (1991) Insufficient dietary carbohydrate during training does it impair performance? *International Journal of Sport Nutrition* **1**, 28–44.

Stanely, W.C., Wisneski, J.A., Gertz, E.W., Neese, R.A. and Brooks, G.A. (1986) Lactate metabolism in exercising human skeletal muscle: evidence for lactate extraction during net lactate release. *Journal of Applied Physiology* **60**, 1116–1120.

Wasserman, K. Whipp, B.J., Koyal, S.N. & Beaver, W.L. (1973) Anaerobic threshold and respiratory gas exchange during exercise. *Journal of Applied Physiology* **35**, 236–243.

Weltman, A. (1995) *The Blood Lactate Response to Exercise. Current Issues in Exercise Science: Monograph Number 4.* Champaign, IL: Human Kinetics.

Chapter 2
Central adaptations: heart, blood, and lung

Joel M. Stager

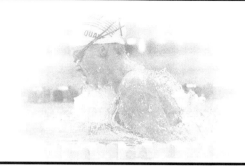

Evolutionary ideas

The model of sport performance that we are working from supposes that the limits to swim performance are multiple and complex. It further proposes that the causes of fatigue are multiple and that the specific factors that allow outstanding performance are dependent upon the nature of the specific event. One conclusion from our discussion in Chapter 1 on energy systems is that the respiratory chain, the transport of oxygen from room air to the mitochondria, may be a limiting factor to performance in events that last beyond several minutes. And yet, the specific limit to aerobic metabolism might be shared across all of the possible parameters that contribute to the respiratory chain rather than any one single parameter (Fig. 2.1).

From the perspective of training theory and an explanation of the underlying physiological mechanisms that confer performance, several concepts need to be considered. The first topic pertains to "symmorphosis," a viable concept to consider in this context and one that is gaining wide acceptance by physiologists.

Symmorphosis

Symmorphosis supposes that within a biological organism, it is difficult (if not impossible) to evolve physiological systems that are limitless in capacity relative to the capacities of other systems in the body. The design of the components in a healthy physiological system is such that it matches the components quantitatively to the functional demands placed upon them. In simple words, current theory suggests that there is no single limiting factor to cardiorespiratory performance, just as no physiological trait can be shown to have a limitless "reserve." Evolution of a trait such that it exists widely in a population requires many thousands of years and some selective advantage. There is no way to maintain a trait, from the evolutionary perspective, if it has no adaptive advantage. That is, if a trait is never exploited as an adaptive advantage, there is no way this trait can be maintained within the gene pool. There are no "limitless" systems.

Because of this, a negative change in the capacity of *any specific link* in the chain, more likely than not, will subsequently act to limit performance. For example, restricted ventilation because of asthma will cause performance to suffer in a meet and in swim practice. This does not necessarily mean that ventilation is *the* limiting factor. Increased ventilation (above normal values) will not necessarily enhance performance because this improvement does not necessarily influence any of the other processes in the oxygen transport chain that also act to limit performance. Matched capacities of the various important physiological processes seem to exist. It now appears to physiologists that all components of a system have about the same maximal ability, "enough but not too much," to perform intensive exercise. All systems reach their maximum capacity at about the same time in a progressively increasing work bout.

Symmorphosis can be expanded to suppose that the adaptations to intensive swim training should be

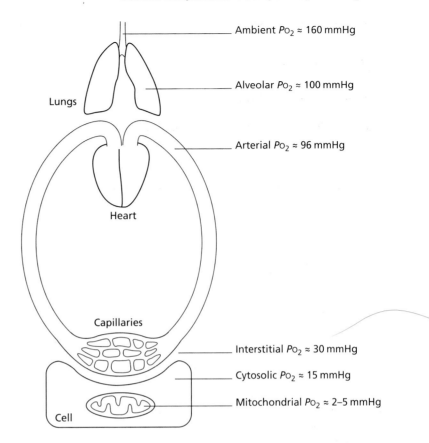

Ambient $P_{O_2} \approx 160$ mmHg

Alveolar $P_{O_2} \approx 100$ mmHg

Lungs

Arterial $P_{O_2} \approx 96$ mmHg

Heart

Capillaries

Interstitial $P_{O_2} \approx 30$ mmHg

Cytosolic $P_{O_2} \approx 15$ mmHg

Mitochondrial $P_{O_2} \approx 2$–5 mmHg

Cell

Fig. 2.1 Elements of the oxygen transport chain include ventilation of air into the lungs, diffusion of gases from alveoli to lung capillaries, convection of blood through the vascular tree, and diffusion of gas across the capillary into the cell and mitochondria. The approximate partial pressure of oxygen (P_{O_2}) is listed for each level of the chain.

appropriate and integrated such that all of the adaptations to training are consistent with the desired outcome of a specific improved performance. Evolution insures, and the theory of symmorphosis implies, that physiological systems are generally well matched in their capacities. Exclusive focus on one specific system might simply be a waste of an athlete's time as improvements in performance can only be achieved through improvements in each of the specifically linked and carefully matched processes. Although not specifically advertised as such, Jan Olbrecht's recent reinterpretation of the meaning of the lactic acid profiles in the blood of swimmers is consistent with the "symmorphosis" theory. Changes in the blood lactic acid threshold may be related to changes in aerobic capacity, or to changes in the capacity of the anaerobic systems, or changes in both. Improvements in performance come as a result of improvements in multiple components in carefully matched systems.

Weak link theory

The competing hypothesis (and much older theory) suggests that one physiological system may fail much sooner than any of the others and training should specifically focus on this "fatal" weakness. For lack of a more sophisticated term, we will call this the "weak link" theory. Central to this theory is the idea that certain physiological systems have measurable and considerable reserves and others do not. A reserve is defined as the capacity of any given component— cardiac, vascular, pulmonary, etc—above that which is required during maximal exercise. In this theory, when an athlete is engaged in an intensive exercise bout, his or her limit is set by the "weakest link," or rather that system with the smallest reserve. When the capacity of the system with the smallest reserve is exhausted, the ability to continue to exercise, or rather the ability to increase or sustain exercise, no longer exists. The swimmer becomes exhausted, or reaches the point of fatigue. Physiologists have long searched for the weak link limiting aerobic capacity. This search has been largely to no avail and no consensus among scientists has been reached as to what physiological component represents the weak link. Consistent with the concept of symmorphosis, no weak link should be identifiable. The inability to specifically do so adds further support for this theory.

An example of symmorphosis might have been provided in the early 1920s by the famous automobile industrialist Henry Ford. He is said to have frequented junkyards as a means to determine how well the various parts in his cars performed. When he came across a part that was never broken and never needed replacement, he was said to have ordered it redesigned, as he felt it must have been "overengineered." By "down engineering" the part, it didn't make the car perform any worse, but made the car less expensive, which allowed more people to afford it. Henry reasoned that by the car being less expensive he would eventually sell more cars and make more money. We might conclude therefore that Ford was an advocate of "industrial symmorphosis."

Adaptations to training

It might be helpful to separate morphological or structural adaptations to training from those that are more functional in nature. When a swimmer begins to train, adaptations occur within the various cells, tissues, and systems. These adaptations allow the body to accommodate to the metabolic stress that swim training represents. Some of these adaptations are functional in nature and are outcome variables initiated at the biochemical or cellular level. Some are morphological or structural at the cellular, tissue, or systems level. Functional changes may be considered outcome variables, such as $\dot{V}o_{2max}$ and cardiac output. The structural adaptations are, in theory, the mechanisms by which the functional changes occur. Important structural parameters include heart chamber size, erythrocyte volume, lung surface area, and mitochondrial volume. The importance of mitochondrial volume as a potential contributor to performance was emphasized in Chapter 1. The other three, heart size, erythrocyte volume, and lung surface area, will be dealt with in greater detail in this chapter. The important idea is

that a few key structural improvements lead to important functional outcomes.

Regardless of the nature of the adaptations to swim training, it is clear that in some cases it is the individual bout of exercise that represents the stimulus for adaptation and in other cases it is the cumulative effect of multiple swim training bouts. It is evident that training effects cannot be stored. The effects are a result of what the athlete did rather than what he or she used to do. However, once a trait has reached its capacity to change, there may be a difference between the frequency of training stimulus needed to improve the trait versus the frequency needed to maintain the trait. This is not news.

It is also apparent that many of the training-induced physiological changes occur over considerable time rather than overnight. It is also clear that the nature of the stimulus must be specific, appropriate, and progressive in order for the correct training adaptations to occur. These are well-known tenets of classic training theory—specificity, progression, and adaptation. At the end of the season, the only appropriate structural and functional training adaptations are those that will ultimately lead to improved performance in the individual's targeted event.

It may be, however, that during the swim season, certain outcomes of training are much more general in nature and not specific to the competitive event *per se*. One desirable functional outcome that may only indirectly affect sprint performance, for example, may be quicker recovery from swim competition. Rapid recovery is important, not only from the perspective of being able to withstand subsequent intensive training, but for being able to compete optimally in more than one event per meet. It may be critical for a swimmer to be able to compete well in the morning preliminaries as well as in the evening's finals. Certain structural training responses may also reduce the risk of injury that might subsequently prevent swimmers from performing. The coach needs to keep all of these outcomes in mind when developing an annual swim training plan: being able to recover quickly, remaining injury-free, and being able to perform the target competitive event optimally.

The nature and basis of early season training is largely directed toward central morphological factors—heart, lung, and blood—rather than peripheral factors such as the biochemical characteristics of the skeletal muscle fibers. The ability to pump blood and air across the gas-exchange surface and then convect it to the active muscles is critical in terms of performing work and sustaining it for any length of time. Convective delivery of blood to and from the muscle is critical to the recovery process. Thus early season swim training is usually of lower relative intensity, longer duration, and less specific to the principle competitive swim event.

With that much said it must be pointed out that the nature of the training adaptations will dictate the need and timing of the focus coaches place upon them. For example, structural changes leading toward increased vascularity of the skeletal muscle take considerably greater time than do the biochemical changes that take place within the cell. Increased capillary density is a response that may take many months, if not years, while the majority of the biochemical changes due to training may be fairly complete in a matter of a few months. The increase in vascularity is a response to the needs of the skeletal muscles for nutrients and to the high metabolic rates incurred by the exercise. But the demand for greater delivery is subsequent to the biochemical adaptations that act to increase the demand.

An example might be appropriate in terms of demonstrating the different adaptations that take place. One of the quickest responses to endurance training is an expanded blood volume. A greater blood volume leads to more proficient delivery of blood to the periphery, as well as other positive attributes. The blood volume expansion begins following a single exercise bout. After a week of swim practices, blood volume may increase by 10–15%, with little further increase occurring thereafter. Evidence suggests that the maintenance of these adaptive traits requires much less effort than their original development took. Maintenance may require as few as two or three specific aerobic workouts per week targeted at characteristics inherent in high aerobic capacity.

It has been suggested that as a swimmer travels up the fitness ladder, the hierarchy of performance-limiting factors changes. The heart's ability to pump blood is seen as an early limiting factor, perhaps only secondary to skeletal muscle endurance. As conditioning begins to take place, the increased blood volume and enhanced maximal capacity to pump blood in

large volumes becomes secondary to the ability of the vasculature, for example, to present the blood in close proximity to the muscle cells. Maximal skeletal muscle blood flow is seen as an additional limiting factor in sustained power output. Theoretically, the distance between the capillary and the mitochondria is an additional potentially limiting factor, as this distance will affect the rate of the diffusion of oxygen into the cells.

It is somewhat difficult to determine which occurs first, the need for more oxygen and then the expanded blood volume, capillary density, and cardiac output, or some other sequence of events. But during this time, it is important that the swimmer receives proper nutrition and adequate rest. The changes taking place require tissue building and growth in order to be optimally expressed. Muscle growth and development requires essential amino acid availability. Red blood cell and hemoglobin production require optimal micro- as well as macronutrient intake. While coaches may not be able to change fiber type, they can insure that adaptive responses are optimal by preaching good nutritional practices to their swimmers.

One would suppose, therefore, that the type of training bouts prescribed during the preseason and early season would be those that act to favor aerobic development. These improvements mirror the improvements in the biochemical pathways responsible for aerobic metabolism and those that stimulate an increase in cardiac performance, pulmonary function, and tissue vascularity. We will now look at some of these individual adaptations more closely.

The heart

It is common to consider the human heart as being functionally two hearts, a systemic or left heart and a pulmonary or right heart. The volume demands placed upon the two hearts are similar. When the left heart is required to pump 15 l of blood a minute, the right heart must do so as well because the entire circulation reflects that of a closed system.

The pressure challenges that the two hearts must meet, however, are very different. The left heart must be able to generate pressures well in excess of 200 mmHg, depending upon the flow and resistance

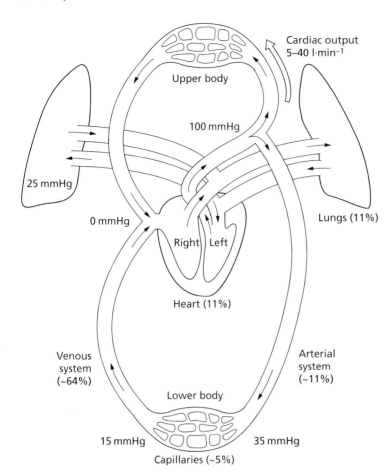

Cardiac output
5–40 l·min⁻¹

Upper body

100 mmHg

25 mmHg

0 mmHg

Lungs (11%)

Right | Left

Heart (11%)

Venous
system
(~64%)

Arterial
system
(~11%)

Lower body

15 mmHg   35 mmHg

Capillaries (~5%)

Fig. 2.2 Elements of the cardiovascular and pulmonary systems with blood pressure and approximate percentage of total blood, i.e., about 64% of the blood is in the systemic veins, 11% each in the heart, lungs, and systemic arteries, and 5% in the capillaries.

characteristics of the active tissues during exercise. The right heart pumps blood to the lungs where pressures rarely exceed 60 mmHg. Because of these pressure differences, the myocardial mass is very different between the right and left ventricles. The right heart is clearly more of a "volume" pump as compared to the left heart, which must work against a considerable pressure load (Fig. 2.2).

Blood flows through the circulation as a function of differences in pressure. The highest pressures must exist in the left ventricle (systolic pressure) and aorta, and then gradually dissipate until nearly zero (relative to ambient tissue pressure) in the right atrium. Venous blood enters the right heart as a result of the pressure being marginally lower (perhaps even slightly negative relative to ambient pressure) than the pressure in the vena cava during the filling phase. The atria act as reservoirs and only minimally assist in

ventricular filling. This atrial assistance may be more important during exercise when filling time becomes limited.

The amount of blood pumped per unit time is referred to as cardiac output and is the product of the number of beats per minute (cardiac frequency) and the volume of blood pumped per beat (stroke volume). During heavy exercise, cardiac output can increase to truly astounding values in athletes with values in the literature exceeding 40 l·min⁻¹. These high volumes are achieved primarily through vascular adjustments improving ventricular filling and increases in stroke volume rather than increases in maximal heart rate.

Cardiac performance is influenced, then, by the volume of the blood in the ventricles prior to contraction (preload) and the resistance that the heart has to overcome during systole (afterload). The vigor of each beat (contractility) also plays a role. Contractility can be affected by internal, inherent factors as well as by external variables such as neural or humeral. All three impact the functional ability of the heart to meet the various metabolic challenges that competitive swimming represents.

Heart size

Johnny Weissmuller, the great Olympian of the early twentieth century, correctly concluded that one of the important traits of a champion swimmer is a large heart. What exactly does "large heart" mean, and how does having a large heart aid performance? Heart size can refer to "chamber size" as well as myocardial thickness. The first reflects the heart's ability to generate flow (volume per unit time) and the second to overcome resistance. Not surprisingly, the evidence suggests that swimmers tend to show both responses to swim training, most likely as a result of the extensive dryland training that is commonly prescribed today and the extensive volume load the swimmers complete while training in the water.

Preload

When athletes train, the characteristics of the training will influence the adaptive responses of the heart. If the athlete is primarily engaged in prolonged, low-intensity exercise, the cardiac adaptations will be a gradual increase in the size of the chambers of the heart, without much change in the thickness of the heart walls. The dimensions of the heart chambers increase in response to stretch or tension. A part of this dimensional increase is due to expanded blood volume. Increased blood volume affects the filling volume during diastole, which then acts to increase stroke volume. Studies have shown that experimental increases or decreases in blood volume result in proportional increases and decreases in stroke volume.

Chamber size affects the volume of the blood that can be pumped with each beat (stroke volume). It is also true, however, that the volume within the chamber will subsequently affect the myocardial contraction through what is known as the Frank–Starling mechanism. Because swimmers are in the prone or supine position while swimming, venous return (blood returning to the heart in the veins) is enhanced as a result of the elimination of the effects of gravity. Increased preload by increased diastolic filling results in stronger myocardial contraction. Stroke volume increases because of increased filling and simultaneously increased emptying.

The heart of an endurance swimmer can be argued to be more efficient when compared on a "metabolic cost per volume of blood pumped per unit time" basis because heart rate and mean arterial pressure are lower at any given exercise intensity. Endurance swim training increases the volume of blood pumped and does so without affecting blood pressure to any great extent. Because the work of the heart can be estimated by multiplying the heart rate by systolic pressure, a reduction in pressure coupled with a slower heart rate means less myocardial work per unit time at a given exercise intensity.

Structural volume changes in the ventricular walls occur as a result of adding myofibrils—in series—to the myocardial cells. In response to chronically altered demands, ventricular size increases, leading to an increase in maximal stroke volume as well as maximal cardiac output. Sedentary individuals exhibit maximal stroke volumes of approximately 135 ml · beat^{-1}, while values reported for highly trained athletes approach 200 ml · beat^{-1}. The importance of this difference cannot be overstressed. From rest to maximal exercise, then, the athlete is able to increase stroke volume by more than 100 ml · beat^{-1} as compared to rest, while the sedentary individual can only increase stroke volume by about 50 ml · beat^{-1}. This represents a tremendous advantage in terms of the amount of blood that can be pumped in a given amount of time. Research has shown that stroke volume increases account for a large portion of the increase in oxygen consumption seen with training.

There is very little evidence to suggest that heart chamber size is an inherited trait. Children show little dimensional variation and twin studies do not support the conclusion of any significant genetic control. It has been suggested that the myocardial sac, the fibrous sheath that surrounds the heart, represents the limit for expanding chamber size. What ultimately determines myocardial sac volume and to what extent it can be increased after physical maturity remain to be identified.

Afterload

Swimming does not induce systolic blood pressures as high as that seen during running or resistance training. The resistance to ventricular emptying, largely represented by mean arterial pressure, is referred to as "afterload." Lower afterload while swimming is thought to exist despite the observation that exercise which requires upper body musculature tends to result in higher pressures than similar exercise using larger lower body muscles. This is because the forces generated are low and swimmers are in the prone or supine positions. In this regard, little attention has been focused upon the habit of swimmers to "catch breath." Swimmers tend to gasp a quick inhalation and then exhale in a controlled, prolonged fashion (relative to inhalation time). This might result in a change to the vascular dynamics of the right heart by affecting right heart afterload. Because of measurement difficulties, however, the availability of data on the pulmonary arterial blood pressure of swimmers while swimming is limited.

Cardiac output

Stroke volume has been suggested to plateau with an increase in exercise intensity. The plateau occurs between 50 and 60% of maximal exercise during upright exercise. Further increases in cardiac output are then thought to be a result of increases in heart rate. Recent evidence in athletes suggests that stroke volume may not plateau in the highly trained and may indeed increase up until maximum exercise. This may partially account for the increased cardiac output observed in the highly trained endurance athletes and be permissive to the increased rate of aerobic metabolism.

Early research on the effects of training on the heart concluded that exercise lasting 2–5 min in duration was effective as a means to increase heart chamber volume and thus stroke volume. Interestingly, the focus of much of this research was on the interval of rest that was optimal rather than the interval of exercise that was best. The conclusion of this work seemed to suggest that rest intervals allowing heart rate to return to values around 120 beats$\cdot$min^{-1} were most effective in producing favorable cardiac adaptations. The specific rest interval was a function of the athletes'

responses rather than a set time interval. As the athletes increased their level of fitness, the rest interval shortened to accommodate the improvements in recovery rate. While this is a very old concept dating back to the early 1900s, there have recently been suggestions of a return to this "recovery based" training model as a more effective means to bring about positive individualistic adaptive training responses.

What is the advantage of the heart being able to pump more blood? Some researchers believe that skeletal muscle blood flow is actually the most important limit to aerobic metabolism. If blood flow to the muscles is mechanically increased beyond its natural limit, it has been shown in isolated muscle that its aerobic capacity can be elevated. On the whole organism level, there is a very high correlation between aerobic capacity and the maximal volume of blood the heart can pump in a minute. Exercise in the heat, which diverts blood flow to the skin for thermoregulatory purposes, is shown to depress aerobic capacity. It has even been suggested that the ventilatory muscles compete with the locomotor muscles during heavy exercise and effectively compete for a portion of the limited cardiac output. Maximal cardiac output, thus, may be the single best predictor of maximal aerobic capacity.

While heart rate can modulate cardiac output, differences in stroke volume play the more significant role during intensive exercise. Swimmers hoping to compete in the longer competitive events, such as the 400-m events and beyond, require sustained high rates of metabolism such that a high aerobic capacity is certainly an advantage, if not a requirement. Thus, cardiac output may be a permissive trait that allows for a high aerobic capacity and thus exceptional endurance performance. Cardiac output should be considered a central, functional limitation to maximal aerobic metabolism. Sprinters have much less need and much less capacity for aerobic adaptations. Thus, aerobic capacity becomes only of secondary importance to sprint performance, serving primarily as a means of improving recovery time.

Substrate delivery

The current view is that during exercise, both carbohydrate and lipid transport from the capillary into the muscle cells reach a maximal rate at moderate exercise intensities. Beyond these modest levels, then, the mitochondria must rely upon intramuscular fuel sources. It is tempting to conclude that metabolic substrate delivery might be a limiting factor for metabolism. However, the rate at which pyruvate can be supplied to the mitochondria does not appear to be limited above and beyond the capacity of the mitochondria to oxidize it. Limiting factors to fatty acid metabolism are not as well understood, with β-oxidation and transfer of fatty acids to the mitochondrial matrix both being potentially limiting to aerobic metabolism. Regardless, mitochondrial oxidation does not appear to be limited by fuel substrate availability, but rather by the supply of oxygen from the capillaries. This does not discount the importance of mitochondrial volume in this regard. However, oxygen transport is and should be the focus of the discussion pertaining to limiting factors to performance as it plays a crucial role in setting an upper limit to the ability to sustain work.

The demand for increased peripheral blood flow (increased oxygen transport) during exercise resides within the muscles, while at least some degree of co-ordination of this flow resides within the CNS. Thus, as exercise intensity increases, metabolism must go up to match the energy expended to do work. This requires increased gas exchange (functional), an increased gas-exchange surface (structural), and to a lesser extent, increased mobilization of metabolically important substrates. All of these parameters require enhanced delivery, characterized by high flow and an expanded surface area for exchange within the tissues. The focus is on the ability of the heart to deliver this volume, although structural changes within the muscle (capillary density, for example) may also act as limiting factors.

Training responses

It must be kept in mind that the structural adaptations to intensive training described here require substantial amounts of time. These training-induced changes are organic in nature. Many training-induced improvements are based upon physiological adaptations to the stresses imposed by a vigorous training program. They are not learned adaptive responses or simple changes in biomechanical efficiency. Increased vascularity, increased red blood cell volume, and heart wall adaptations require structural changes within

multiple tissues. Adaptations of this nature take time! Researchers have shown that it takes minimally 6–8 weeks of exercise to result in the majority of the increase in the desired aerobic training responses.

Heart rate

Maximal heart rates are not observed to be altered to any great extent by training. Maximal heart rates vary somewhat from day to day, are individualistic, and partially related to inherited traits. Maximum heart rate is a function of the biophysical constraints imposed by the mechanisms that determine firing rates of excitable tissues. There is a refractory period following each heart beat during which the various ions need to be concentrated appropriately across the various cell membranes. In addition, the time required by the spread of the action potential across the myocardium partners to limit the maximal heart rate. Finally, there is a certain amount of time needed for ventricular filling. As hearts approach and exceed 200 beats $\cdot$ min^{-1}, the end diastolic volume becomes less, resulting in no significant advantage in terms of further increases in cardiac output. Maximal values for mature swimmers range from 185 beats $\cdot$ min^{-1} to values over 200. Smaller, younger swimmers tend to have higher heart rates, possibly as a function of a smaller heart mass and a shorter conduction distance.

The results of cross-sectional observations consistently show a decline in maximal heart rate with increasing age. However, this relationship might vary as a function of lifestyle. Master swimmers who have maintained intensive, daily habitual physical activity tend to show less decline with age when compared to the age-related changes reported for the general population.

As a swimmer becomes better conditioned, early morning, resting heart rate is observed to decline. The mechanism is referred to as "parasympathetic overtone" and has a biophysical mechanism. Acetylcholine released at the end plates of the vagus nerve acts to slow the spontaneous firing rate of the pacemaker cells of the SA node. Resting heart rates less than 50 beats $\cdot$ min^{-1} are not uncommon in well-conditioned endurance athletes. Increases in early morning heart rate may be an early symptom of an inability to adequately recover from the preceding workout. It may also warn against impending overtraining.

The rise in heart rate reflects the involvement of the sympathetic nervous system in response to the stress imposed by training.

Heart rate has been used for many years as an index of exercise intensity. Individual differences in heart rate and daily fluctuations make its use somewhat of an art rather than a science. The "truthfulness" of the athlete, meaning the accuracy of self-reported postexercise heart rates, may also limit the usefulness of heart rate as a measure of relative exercise intensity. Daily fluctuations may be in the 2–3 beats $\cdot$ min^{-1} range at any given exercise intensity. When beats are counted per 10 s, as is usually done, a missed beat (or added beat) will result in an additional 6-beat difference when reported as a minute value. The rapid postexercise decline in heart rate also may influence the estimated exercise heart rate. A range of heart rate values with a fairly broad spread is thus appropriate.

The blood

The concentration of hemoglobin within the blood plays a leading role in transport of gases to and from the active tissues. As noted earlier, blood volume expansion has a direct mechanical effect upon stroke volume through increased venous filling and the Frank–Starling effect. Blood volume expansion may also impact venous compliance and central venous pressure, acting in concert to assist right heart venous return. Increases in venous return represent equivalent increases in cardiac output.

The increase in blood volume may additionally act as a buffer against reductions in cardiac performance because of a loss of vascular volume resulting from sweating. Although swimmers are not conscious of it, sweating occurs during swim training, particularly when water temperatures are high. Coaches should be conscious of this and cognizant of scenarios in which the athletes can become dehydrated or hypohydrated. A simple pre- to post-workout weight comparison, particularly when training in warm water above 80° F, will demonstrate the magnitude of this effect.

Just as important as the volume increases are the increases in the ability of the blood to carry oxygen. This is the second "structural" adaptation (in addition to heart chamber size) that acts to enhance aerobic

metabolism. Increased O_2-carrying capacity will have a proportional increase in the transport of oxygen to the periphery. The key component of this is the complex molecule hemoglobin and its capacity to reversibly bind to oxygen.

Hemoglobin

It is evident that changes in the concentration of hemoglobin ([Hb]) result in proportional changes in O_2 delivered to the peripheral tissues. Decreases in the amount of oxygen bound to hemoglobin (arterial saturation), such as those caused by altitude (hypobaric hypoxia), lung disease (hypoventilation, diffusion limitation, or ventilation/perfusion mismatch), or perhaps most importantly, smoking cigarettes (an increase in carboxyhemoglobin), will cause decreases in oxygen transport that are directly proportional to the extent of arterial saturation. Any factor that lowers O_2 delivery or the partial pressure of O_2 in the arterial blood will subsequently limit work done by limiting oxygen transport and thus aerobic power output.

Training responses

The structural variables capable of increasing in response to exercise are few and probably limited to increases in stroke volume and [Hb]. The usual pattern with training is a rapid plasma volume expansion with little effective increase in [Hb]. Endurance-trained athletes are observed to express "pseudoanemia" as a result. Nevertheless, athletes participating in extensive training should be monitored for adequate iron intake and body iron stores.

Hemoglobin production

Poor nutrition can impact hemoglobin production and adversely affect the replacement of aging erythrocytes. Because mature erythrocytes do not contain a nucleus or DNA, they have a finite viability on the order of 120 days. The complexity of hemoglobin is such that poor nutrition can affect hemoglobin production in several ways. The common outcome is anemia and a decline in total erythrocyte volume. The importance of this cannot be overstated and the routine screening of elite performers as a means of diagnosis and prevention is warranted.

Altitude training has been proposed for years as a means to initiate functional changes by inducing structural improvements in erythrocyte volume. The justification for this is associated with proposed increases in [Hb]. However, the scientific literature, in general, does not support altitude training as an effective means of improving subsequent sea-level performance. Nevertheless, the attitude of many coaches is that altitude has not necessarily been shown to be detrimental to performance—so what is the risk? The physiologists counter that the risks are associated with limited peripheral adaptations because the altitude training intensity must be adjusted downward to account for the limited oxygen transport. Although there has been recent research presented upon a "live high, train low" training regime for endurance runners, convincing evidence is limited and the practicality for swimming is questioned.

The lung

There do not appear to be many structural changes that specifically occur in the lung in response to intensive training. This has led to the suggestion that the lung may be "built in excess" to accommodate heavy exercise. Other training-induced improvements in the more plastic elements of the oxygen transport chain simply "catch up" to the lungs. The muscles responsible for ventilation, however, certainly increase their endurance, similar to the locomotive muscles used for swimming. There is only limited evidence for other training-induced adaptations.

Similar to athletes in other sports, the lungs of swimmers have not been shown to grow larger in response to training when normal growth and development are accounted for. The surface area for gas exchange in the lung is thus fixed once adult stature is attained. Nevertheless, swimmers have been reported to have lungs that are comparatively larger than age- and height-matched sedentary controls. It has not been possible to determine if this is an adaptation to prolonged swim training or perhaps a selective trait that allows for swimming success. Cross-sectional research has simply shown that in contrast to other highly trained athletes, when matched for height, swimmers have comparatively larger lungs. In terms of functional

implications, it is uncertain if this is an advantage to the swimmer as far as gas exchange is concerned, or perhaps the larger volume of gas in the chest simply improves buoyancy.

The lungs represent the interface between the environment and the blood inside the vasculature. They have evolved as an efficient gas-exchange surface. In a healthy lung, it takes less than a third of a second for the blood returning from the active tissues to equilibrate with the gases in the lung. At rest, the transit time of blood in the lung approximates three quarters of a second. Thus, there is plenty of "exchange" time to spare. This reserve is reduced during exercise and the extent of the decline in transit time is related to maximal cardiac output. Recent research suggests that in highly trained runners, cardiac output may be so great that the time available for complete equilibration in the lung may be inadequate. This sets up a secondary diffusion limitation such that arterial oxygenation may be less than normal during very heavy work. Currently, there is no evidence showing similar limitations in swimmers.

The swimmer's lung

Interestingly, enhanced pulmonary diffusion capacities have been demonstrated in swimmers at rest as well as during exercise. It is unclear if this is related to the larger area for gas exchange, more even gas exchange within the lung, or due to some other adaptation. Diffusion capacity for O_2 across the alveolar–capillary membrane is determined by the following structural parameters: alveolar and capillary surface area, the thickness of the membrane and plasma layer separating the erythrocyte from the endothelium, and pulmonary capillary blood volume.

The observation of greater diffusion capacity in swimmers is consistent even when diffusion capacity is adjusted for body size and total lung capacity. It has been suggested that alveolar hypertrophy or hyperplasia may account for the differences observed, yet no direct evidence exists for either of these two possibilities in swimmers. There exists limited, yet intriguing, evidence for dysanaptic growth in the lung of swimmers favoring increases in alveolar mass over increases in growth within the conducting zones of the lung.

A further hypothesis pertaining to the differences observed between swimmers and others supposes that the early intensive training that swimmers perform is responsible for the observed pulmonary adaptations. The literature consistently shows that successful swimmers begin training, on the average, somewhere between 8 and 9 years of age. This compares to data obtained from athletes in other sports that show most athletes begin training in an organized fashion between 14 and 15 years of age. There is no direct evidence to support early training as the cause of the pulmonary differences discussed, but at least one training study using immature rats suggests that early training might be causal in nature to lung adaptations observed in competitive swimmers.

Ventilation

The ventilatory muscles of the chest and the diaphragm act to keep the lung ventilated in a tightly coordinated manner in response to changes in blood gases. The goal is to keep the composition of gas in the lung constant (and thus arterial gases constant) regardless of the metabolism of the tissues. If more O_2 is removed from the lung gas by the blood, then more air must be ventilated to keep the gas composition in the lung constant. That is not to imply that lung gases are monitored by the central nervous system, although this has been proposed at various times in history. It simply is meant to imply how tightly the system is regulated.

Ventilation is controlled such that as exercise intensity increases, pulmonary ventilation increases proportional to the intensity of exercise. As exercise becomes more intense, however, there exists an intensity beyond which ventilation increases at an even greater rate. While this has been described for runners and cyclists, the process is much more complicated in swimmers because of their activity taking place in the water. The importance of this increase is severalfold.

First, the significance of the increase is related to concurrent increases in cardiac output. Because ventilation can increase to a greater extent than cardiac output, the ratio of the two increases as exercise intensity increases. The outcome of this is an increase in alveolar oxygen partial pressure, lower alveolar CO_2, and a more favorable environment for diffusion. Because swimmers exercise in the prone or supine position, it is also suggested that the postural effects upon blood flow in the lung might not exist, resulting in more homogeneous ventilation versus perfusion match from the base to the apex of the lung. Both mechanisms would act to insure that arterial saturation is maintained during intensive exercise.

Second, with the increase in ventilation being proportionally greater than the increase in metabolism, there is an increase in the elimination of CO_2 from the tissues and lung. Because of the way in which CO_2 is transported from the tissues, increased ventilation will act to buffer the changes in acidity by the elimination of CO_2 in the lung.

With the possible exception of the backstroke, ventilation during swimming requires an artificial breathing pattern in the sense that breathing is restricted by elements demanded by stroke mechanics. Swimmers might therefore be described as using an "obligatory controlled frequency breathing" pattern. The breathing frequency of a swimmer is "entrained" to the pull frequency of the various strokes. The swimmer unconsciously regulates ventilatory volumes by increasing the size of each breath (tidal volume) or by increasing the breathing frequency through increased stroke tempo. This happens because swimmers can breathe only when their faces are in a position to do so. Recent evidence proposes that swimmers exhibit similar pulmonary traits as runners who have engaged in specific inspiratory muscle training.

Breathing patterns

One of the biggest problems coaches fight is young swimmers who modify their stroke pattern in order to accommodate their breathing. Rather than learning to breathe when optimal (in terms of having the least effect upon their propulsive movements), many beginning swimmers allow breathing to completely dictate their stroke characteristics. It is not uncommon to see experienced swimmers even "overbreathe" or take breaths because of habit, when no breath is actually needed. Swimmers breathe habitually according to a rhythmic cadence that seems, at times, to override physiological cues. This is not common, or perhaps not as obvious, during other modes of exercise, but from the coach's view, is a hard habit to break in swimming.

Because of the difficulty of measuring breathing parameters while actually swimming, not much is known about the specifics of breathing strategies of swimmers. For instance, little is known about the ability of a swimmer to maintain blood gases while swimming. If the swimmer reduces the frequency at which a breath is taken (i.e., intermittent breath holding or "hypoxic" training), does alveolar ventilation suffer to the extent that arterial blood saturation drops and CO_2 levels rise? Some evidence exists which suggests that under certain circumstances they may. This would seem logical particularly in the well-trained endurance swimmer who is already working at the limits of the oxygen transport system.

Another interesting topic to consider is the effect of bilateral breathing on blood gases. Bilateral breathing refers to the swimmer breathing during the crawl stroke in a pattern that alternates from side to side, usually every third stroke. The swimmer might do this as a means to keep an eye on the competition on either side or to "even out" the pull pattern. In eight strokes (right arm, left arm, etc.) a swimmer would usually take four breaths. With bilateral breathing, a swimmer might take only three or two. The decrease in breathing frequency would be expected to be of little physiological significance as long as the swimmer can expand the size of each breath. Swimmers' breathing rates approximate 30 breaths $\cdot$ min^{-1}, which may be less than half of that observed in athletes while running at a quick training pace. It is possible for the swimmer to increase breathing frequency by simply increasing stroke tempo. A quicker stroke tempo is not necessarily a bad thing unless the swimmer does so by shortening each stroke. It would seem that for short events, those where power output is most significant, the swimmer might be better off simply breathing to the normal or dominant side.

Breath holding

Breath holding has been an issue in swimming for some time. In the present context, breath holding will refer specifically to the cessation of breathing beyond some usual breakpoint rather than breathing using some slightly reduced frequency (hypoventilation). Both breath holding and reduced frequency breathing are used as training techniques in swimming. The opposite practice of hyperventilating as a means to blow off CO_2 and thus increase the time for a breath hold is also commonplace within competitive swimming. This maneuver is relatively uncommon prior to

competitive events (except perhaps in the shortest sprints) but all too common during practice sessions.

The problem with hyperventilation followed by a breath hold lies in the rapid reduction in arterial O_2 that occurs with intensive exercise while breath holding. Breathing is regulated in part by the partial pressures of gases within the blood. When swimmers hyperventilate, they lower arterial CO_2, thus eliminating what is the strongest stimulus to breath. Hyperventilation has little effect upon arterial O_2, however, as the blood is normally very nearly saturated with oxygen. In response to breath holding then, the drive to breathe has been eliminated and the athletes swim underwater as far and as fast as they can. Because metabolism is increased, large amounts of O_2 are extracted from the blood in a single pass through the circulatory system. If no breaths have been taken, upon the blood's return to the lung for gas exchange, no new O_2 is available, and thus blood O_2 drops. The rapid and drastic drop in O_2 can act as a CNS depressant and can rapidly cause a loss of consciousness. This occurs because the brain has little to no metabolic ability to produce energy without oxygen. The outcome may be fatal if the swimmer passes out with no witnesses to take him or her out of the water. Because breathing has stopped owing to the depressed CNS activity, it may be difficult to initiate breathing even if the swimmer is now on the pool deck. This practice is extremely unwise and provides no benefit to the swimmer in terms of desired training adaptations.

Controlled frequency breathing (hypoxic training)

The idea behind reducing breathing frequency is related to the idea that exposure to lower O_2 pressures has a beneficial effect upon muscular adaptations. It was hypothesized that capillary density, muscle myoglobin levels, and mitochondrial mass may be increased. In short, the idea was that controlled frequency breathing (CFB, or intermittent breath holding) would result in training responses similar to those seen during altitude exposure. The debate, however, has always been whether or not CFB results in hypoxia or just hypercapnea (elevated CO_2). Again, the difficulty in determining which is the case is related to the difficulty in collecting measurements in the water. Given the recent data obtained from runners, however, it seems likely that intermittent breath hold-ing must result in O_2 desaturation if gas exchange in the lung is disturbed. Limited data from swimmers suggest that alveolar gases can be altered significantly by CFB but the exercise bout may have to extend be-yond 2 min and the exercise intensity must be main-tained at high levels. These conditions relate to the gradual decline in alveolar gases that occurs during this relative hypoventilation until the diffusion time required for mixed venous blood to equilibrate with alveolar gases is insufficient. What remains to be deter-mined is whether or not there is any beneficial effect of this brief, intermittent hypoxemia upon competitive swim performance.

Snorkel training

A corollary to CFB is the use by swimmers of snorkels while completing interval sets. The effect of a snorkel is essentially enlargement of the volume of the anatomi-cal dead space within the lung. This makes it necessary for the swimmer to increase the depth of breathing to overcome the added volume from the snorkel. When the swimmer inhales, the first air to reach the lung is the air inside the snorkel. This air includes the air exhaled from the prior breath. In order to ventilate the lung with fresh air, the swimmer must increase the depth of each breath to overcome the volume of air contained within the snorkel. Until breathing vol-ume or ventilatory mechanics can be shown to be a limiting factor in swim performance, this should be considered yet another coaching practice that is lit-tle more than another way to teach the swimmer to tolerate excessive pain and suffering.

Summary

Coaching success results from the induction of opti-mal training adaptations in the existent physiologi-cal makeup of the swimmer. The important param-eters are numerous and can roughly be divided into structural and functional variables. The functional adaptations generally come as a result of underlying structural improvements. Because the limitations to the various "links in the oxygen transport chain" are generally well matched, improvements are a result of

proportional changes in multiple steps rather than improvements in one "weak link." Stroke volume in-creases as a result of morphological increases in ven-tricular volume and blood volume. This leads to an increase in cardiac output, which is highly correlated with increases in aerobic capacity.

Mitochondrial metabolic activity ultimately sets the demand for substrates and oxygen transport. This is masked, however, by the limits set by the cardiopul-monary system's ability to "deliver" during very in-tensive, prolonged exercise. The ability to sustain in-tensive exercise fueled largely by aerobic metabolism is a function of the match between this high tis-sue demand and the abilities of the delivery system to meet them. For elite endurance performance this match is everything. As we shall see in the next chap-ter, however, for the sprinter success lies in the abil-ity of the peripheral tissues to generate propulsive power.

Recommended reading

Adams, T.D., Yanowitz, F.G., Fischer, A.G., Ridges, J.D., Nelson, A.G., Hagen, A.D., Williams, R.R. & Hunt, S.C. (1985) Heritability of cardiac size: an echocardiographic study of monozygotic and dizygotic twins. *Circulation* **71**, 39–44.

Andrew, G.M., Becklake, M.R., Guleria, J.S. & Bates, D.V. (1972) Heart and lung functions in swimmers and non-athletes during growth. *Journal of Applied Physiology* **32**, 245–251.

Astrand, P.O. & Saltin, B. (1961) Maximal oxygen uptake and heart rate in various types of muscular activity. *Journal of Applied Physiology* **16**, 977–981.

Barclay, J.K. & Stainsby, W.N. (1975) The role of blood flow in limiting maximal metabolic rate in muscle. *Medicine and Science in Sports and Exercise* **7**, 116–119.

Bevegard, S., Holmgren, A. & Johnson, B. (1963) Circulatory studies in well trained athletes at rest and during heavy exercise with special reference to stroke volume and in-fluence of body position. *Acta Physiologica Scandinavica* **57**, 26–50.

Bielen, E., Fagard, R. & Amery, A. (1990) Inheritance of heart structure and exercise capacity: a study of left ventric-ular structure and exercise capacity in 7-year-old twins. *European Heart Journal* **11**, 7–16.

Bradley, P.W., Troup, J. & vanHandel, P.J. (1985) Pulmonary function measurements in US elite swimmers. *Journal of Swimming Research* **2**, 23–28.

Bryne-Quinn, E., Weil, J.V., Sodal, I., Fillez, G.F. & Grover, R.F. (1971) Ventilatory control in the athlete. *Journal of Applied Physiology* **30**, 91–99.

Colan, S.D. (1997) Mechanics of left ventricular systolic and diastolic function in physiological hypertrophy of the athlete's heart. *Cardiology Clinics* **15**, 355–372.

Cordain, L. & Stager, J. (1988) Pulmonary structure and function in swimmers. *Sports Medicine* **6**, 271–278.

Coyle, E.F., Hopper, M.K. & Coggan, A.R. (1990) Maximal oxygen uptake relative to plasma expansion. *International Journal of Sports Medicine* **11**, 116–119.

Dempsey, J.A. (1986) Is the lung built for exercise? *Medicine and Science in Sports and Exercise* **18**, 143–155.

Dempsey, J.A., Hanson, P.G. & Henderson, K.S. (1984) Exercise induced hypoxemia in healthy human subjects at sea level. *Journal of Physiology (London)* **355**, 161–175.

diPrampero, P.E. (1985) Metabolic and circulatory limitation to VO₂max at the whole animal level. *Journal of Experimental Biology* **115**, 319–332.

Eichner, E.R. (1992) Sports anemia, iron supplements and blood doping. *Medicine and Science in Sports and Exercise* **24**, S315–S318.

Engstrom, I., Ericksson, B.O., Karlberg, P., Lundin, A., Saltin, B. *et al.* (1978) Long term effect of previous swim training in girls: ten year follow-up of the "girl swimmer." *Acta Paediatrica Scandinavica* **67**, 285–292.

Fu, F.H. (1976) The effects of physical training on the lung growth of infant rates. *Medicine and Science in Sports and Exercise* **8**, 226–229.

Gehr, P., Mwangi, D.K., Amman, A., Maloiy, G.M.O., Taylor, R.C. & Weibel, E.R. (1981) Design of the mammalian respiratory system. V. Scaling morphometric pulmonary diffusing capacity to body mass: wild and domestic animals. *Respiration Physiology* **44**, 61–86.

Gleser, M.A., Horstman, D.H. & Mello, R.P. (1974) The effects on VO₂max of adding arm work to maximal leg work. *Medicine and Science in Sports and Exercise* **6**, 104–107.

Gollnick, P.D. & Saltin, B. (1982) Significance of skeletal oxidative enzyme enhancement with endurance training. *Clinical Physiology* **2**, 1–12.

Holloszy, J.O. & Booth, F.W. (1976) Biochemical adaptation to endurance exercise in muscle. *Annual Review of Physiology* **38**, 273–291.

Holmer, I. & Gullstrand, L. (1980) Physiological responses to swimming with a controlled frequency of breathing. *Scandinavian Journal of Sports Science* **2**, 1–6.

Holmgren, A. & Astrand, P.O. (1966) Pulmonary diffusing capacity and the dimensions and functional capacities of the oxygen transport system in humans. *Journal of Applied Physiology* **21**, 1463–1470.

Hoppeler, H., Lüthi, P., Claassen, H., Weibel, E.R. & Howald, H. (1973) The ultrastructure of the normal human skeletal muscle. A morphometric analysis on untrained men, women and well-trained orienteers. *Pflügers Archiv* **344**, 217–232.

Hoppeler, H., Mathieu, O., Krauer, R., Claassen, H., Armstrong, R.B. & Weibel, E.R. (1981) Design of the mammalian respiratory system. VI. Distribution of mitochondria and capillaries in various muscles. *Respiration Physiology* **44**, 87–111.

Hoppeler, H. & Weibel, E.R. (1998) Limits for oxygen and substrate transport in mammals. *Journal of Experimental Biology* **201**, 1051–1064.

Jones, J.H. & Lindstedt, S.L. (1993) Limits to maximal performance. *Annual Review Physiology* **55**, 547–569.

Jones, J.H., Longworth, K.E., Lindholm, A., Conley, K.E., Karas, R.H., Kayar, S.K. & Taylor, C.R. (1989) Oxygen transport during exercise in large mammals. I. Adaptive variation in oxygen demand. *Journal of Applied Physiology* **67**, 862–870.

Klieber, M. (1961) *The Fire of Life: An Introduction to Animal Energetics*. New York: Wiley, p. 454.

Leith, D.E. & Bradley, M.E. (1976) Ventilatory muscle strength and endurance. *Journal of Applied Physiology* **41**, 508–516.

Levine, B.D. & Stray-Gunderson, J. (1997) Living high-training low: effect of moderate altitude acclimatization with low altitude training on performance. *Journal of Applied Physiology* **83**, 102–112.

Lindstedt, S.L. & Conley, K.E. (2001) Human aerobic performance: too much ado about limits to VO₂. *Journal of Experimental Biology* **204**, 3195–3199.

Lindstedt, S.L., Wells, D.J., Jones, J.H., Hoppeler, H. & Thronsom, H.A. (1988) Limitation to aerobic performance in mammals: interaction of structure and demand. *International Journal of Sports Medicine* **9**, 210–217.

Margulis, L. (1981) *Symbiosis in Cell Evolution*. San Francisco: Freeman.

Morgan, H.E. & Baker, K.E. (1991) Cardiac hypertrophy mechanical neural and endocrine dependence. *Circulation* **83**, 13–25.

Newman, R., Smalley, B.F. & Thomson, M.L. (1961) A comparison between body size and lung function of swimmers and normal school children. *Journal of Physiology (London)* **156**, 9–10.

Reuschlein, P.S., Reddan, W.G., Burpee, J., Gee, J.B.L. & Rankin, J. (1968) Effect of physical training on the pulmonary diffusing capacity during submaximal work. *Journal of Applied Physiology* **24**, 152–158.

Saltin, B. & Strange, S. (1992) Maximal oxygen uptake: "'old" and "new" arguments for a cardiovascular limitation. *Medicine and Science in Sports and Exercise* **24**, 30–37.

Shapiro, L.M. (1997) The morphological consequences of systemic training. *Cardiology Clinics* **15**, 373–379.

Smith, M.L., Hudson, D.L., Graitzer, H.M. & Raven, P.B. (1989) Exercise training bradycardia: the role of autonomic balance. *Medicine and Science in Sports and Exercise* **21**, 40–44.

Taylor, C.R., Karas, R.H., Weibel, E.R. & Hoppeler, H. (1987) Adaptive variation in the mammalian respiratory system in relation to energetic demand. II. Reaching the limits to oxygen flow. *Respiration Physiology* **69**, 7–26.

Taylor, C.R. & Weibel, E.R. (1981) Design of the mammalian respiratory system. I. Problem and strategy. *Respiration Physiology* **44**, 1–10.

Wagner, P.D., Hoppeler, H. & Saltin, B. (1977) Determinants of maximal oxygen uptake. In: R.G. Crystal, J.B. West, E.R. Weibel & P.J. Barnes, eds. *The Lung, Scientific Foundation*, Vol. 2, 2nd edn. Philadelphia: Lippincott-Raven Publishers, pp. 2033–2041.

Weibel, E.R., Taylor, C.R. & Hoppeler, H. (1991) The concept of symmorphosis: a testable hypothesis of structure–function relationship. *Proceedings of the National Academy of Sciences of the United States of America* **88**, 10357–10361.

Chapter 3
Peripheral adaptations: the skeletal muscles

Joel M. Stager

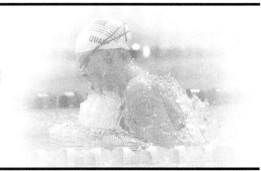

Introduction: sprint vs. endurance

The fastest swimmers in the water are clearly the 50-m freestylers, while the swimmers with the most endurance, i.e., the ability to swim fast for a long time, are the open-water "marathon" swimmers. In order to sprint, the muscles of locomotion need to be able to generate very high mechanical power outputs, but only for short periods of time. In contrast, when swimming distance events, the limb musculature must be able to produce much less peak power, yet sustain relatively moderate power output for a long period of time. Sprinters must train so they can develop a high peak muscular power output, while distance swimmers train so they can sustain power output for extended time periods with little muscular fatigue. Because the events are different, do athletes prepare differently? Are their physiological differences a result of how they train? Or, are the athletes best suited for these contrasting events genetically different?

The answer to these questions is that their abilities are, in part, related to inherent traits exhibited by their peripheral tissues, *and*, in part, to how the athletes prepare for their respective competition. It is important to recognize that regardless of how an athlete is trained, there are inherent differences in the muscular characteristics of talented sprinters and talented distance swimmers. Other differences become apparent in response to drastically different training programs, but many of the essential characteristics common to great sprinters or great endurance athletes are inherited.

Fundamental differences in specific traits of the peripheral tissues, primarily the skeletal muscles, effectively discriminate between great sprinters and talented distance swimmers.

This chapter reviews the characteristics of skeletal muscles and focuses upon those traits that convey specific sprint and endurance swim performance. The later sections of this chapter will integrate this information with the energetic and cardiopulmonary adaptations that must occur in order to provide for elite swim performance in sprint and endurance events.

Muscle anatomy

Anatomically, a muscle, such as the tricep, is composed of distinct, visually discernable units referred to as muscle fascicles (Fig. 3.1). The fascicles are further composed of individual microscopic muscle cells, synonymous with the term "muscle fiber." Muscle fibers are large multinucleated cells whose cytoplasm contains contractile myofilaments, high-energy intermediates, soluble proteins, enzymes for metabolism, ribosomes, mitochondria, and substrates such as glycogen and lipids. Muscle fibers are "excitable," and thus their membranes can propagate action potentials and distribute ions selectively. Muscle fibers can vary in length from a few millimeters to tens of centimeters. They express variable abilities to change certain functional traits in response to external cues such as

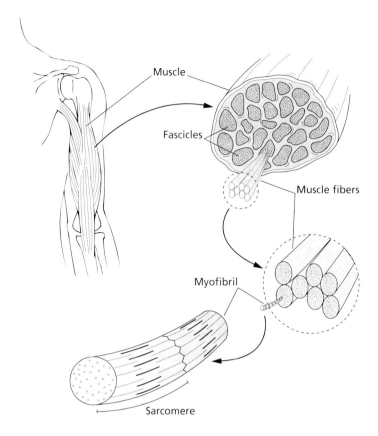

Fig. 3.1 Structural hierarchy of skeletal muscle. Each fascicle contains several muscle fibers. From *Skeletal Muscle Structure, Function, and Plasticity* (ed. R.L. Lieber), 2nd edn, p. 18, 1997, Lippincott Williams & Wilkins, Philadelphia, PA, with zpermission.

the neuroendocrines, nutrition, hypoxia, and exercise. These different adaptive abilities are based upon differences in the muscle's specific genetic makeup.

The myofibrils of a muscle fiber represent nearly 80% of fiber volume (although fibers are perhaps 75% water by weight). The myofibrils contain contractile units, sarcomeres, which are formed by the basic contractile proteins, the myofilaments actin and myosin. Several other important proteins are also present (troponin, tropomyosin, and C-protein) that play important roles in the contractile process (Fig. 3.2). Without going into specific detail, the ability to generate force is related to the interactions between several of these proteins found within the muscle cells. When stimulated to contract by commands sent from the CNS, the force generated by a muscle is related to the chemical bonds formed between these various proteins. Referred to as "cross bridges," the force generated during

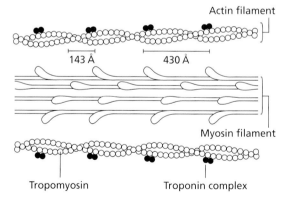

Fig. 3.2 Actin and myosin filaments. Arranged at intervals along the actin filament are the regulatory proteins troponin and tropomyosin. Reproduced with permission from *Skeletal Muscle Structure and Function: Implications for Rehabilitation and Sports Medicine* (ed. R.L. Lieber), 1992, Lippincott Williams & Wilkins, Philadelphia, PA.

a contraction is ultimately a function of the number of bonds or bridges that can collectively be formed.

The limiting factors in terms of force generation are several. First, of course, is cross-sectional muscle area. The greater the cross-sectional area, the more cross bridges in parallel that can be formed. The biophysics of this is complex. The inhibitory protein tropomyosin must be "neutralized" by the release of calcium ions into the muscle cell from special subcellular sites known as the sacroplasmic reticulum. The released calcium binds to troponin, which allows the active sites on actin to form bonds with the active sites on myosin. As this occurs, a ratcheting effect takes place with one myofibril sliding past the other, effectively shortening the fiber. Activation of the contractile complex and maintenance of the muscle membrane's excitability requires ATP, as does the sequestration of the calcium after the muscle contracts. Relaxation, deactivation of the cross bridge, also requires ATP. In short, the contraction of muscle requires energy in the form of ATP in several steps of the process. The limiting factors as far as contraction and relaxation are concerned include several steps that are limited by the availability of ATP. The rates at which these processes can occur are related to the specific activity of the enzymes involved. The extent to which they can occur is related to the metabolic capacity of the muscle fiber. While the force produced and power generated by a muscle are limited by the number of cross bridges that can be formed (or volume of muscle recruited), the ability to sustain a contraction may be limited by the capacities of the metabolic pathways to supply ATP.

Muscular strength and power

Great performances in sprint swim events are related, in part, to the ability of the muscles of locomotion to generate mechanical power. Although the relationship is not necessarily perfect, it is generally true that the greater the muscle mass (greater cross-sectional area), the greater the instantaneous force that can be generated. Bigger muscles can generate more force because they can form more cross bridges within the muscle myofibrils. However, while this sounds fairly simple, the relationship between muscular strength and muscular power is complicated, as is the relationship between muscular power and swim performance.

Strength is related, in part, to the ability of the CNS to recruit muscle fibers and, in part, to muscle cross-sectional area. However, the strongest athletes are not necessarily the fastest swimmers. Recent research suggests that while strength is related to muscular power output in swimmers, strength is not a good predictor of swim performance. This is particularly true for women swimmers. It may be that because women swimmers have less inherent potential to develop muscle mass, they tend to rely on stroke technique and stroke mechanics to generate swim velocity more so than men. Research has shown that when normalized for muscle cross-sectional area, the capacity of muscle to generate force and power is similar for men and women. However, women in general simply have less muscle mass.

Hypertrophy

Organic muscular changes are gained largely through cellular hypertrophy. These improvements occur much more slowly, over many weeks and months. Hypertrophy refers to increases in muscle fiber size by increases in the volume of contractile proteins. There is a suggestion that myogenic or "hypertrophic" changes are more likely to occur in the specific muscle fibers trained, even though increases in the cross-sectional area of all muscle fiber types ultimately contribute to maximal strength gains. There is not much evidence in support of increases in fiber numbers in response to training in humans. Nutrition has been shown to influence the ability of an athlete to induce hypertrophic changes. Limited protein intake (quantity and quality) can limit the anabolic capacity in response to a training program.

The central nervous system

The CNS is also known to play a role in muscular force, muscular power, and muscular fatigue. Initiation of a movement, coordination of the movement, and the generation of the appropriate amount of force required to complete a motor task clearly involves the brain and the spinal cord. There is evidence to suggest that with training, strength and power are, in part, learned skills. Improvements are gained through neurological as well as muscular changes. The neurological changes occur very rapidly and improvements in power can be observed following a single power-training bout. This requires changes within the CNS and peripheral reflex pathways as it occurs too fast to be organic in nature. It is not uncommon to observe increases of 15–20% in power output following one or two power-training sessions.

It has also been shown that the "excitability" of the motor neuron pool within the spinal cord can be an important variable in terms of the amount of force an individual can generate. Research has shown that recovery from extensive training results in an increase in the excitability of the neuron in the spinal cord that correlates to increased power and performance in swimmers.

Fatigue

The cause of muscular fatigue is a very complicated subject. Fatigue can be defined as a decline in the force a muscle can generate. One theory of muscular fatigue is that it is more a function of CNS transmitter depletion than it is an inability of the metabolic pathways to maintain energy supplies within the muscle. The symptoms of Parkinson's disease include a general feeling of fatigue and a need for subjectively greater efforts to complete even minimal muscular tasks. Parkinson's disease is thought to be related to transmitter depletion within specific areas in the brain responsible for initiating movements. Pharmacologic therapies that enhance transmitter production or biological activity reduce the severity of the symptoms of Parkinson's disease, at least in the short term. It is not impossible that overtraining and excessive fatigue in swimmers may be partially mediated by similar mechanisms.

We have seen previously that a cause of fatigue may be metabolic, particularly in short sprint swims. Fatigue can result from a depletion of available energy because of an inhibition of the metabolic pathways. This can be caused by the accumulation of metabolic by-products such as hydrogen ions. This is suggested as one cause of fatigue in very intensive sprint activities. In contrast, fatigue can occur as a result of insufficient substrate availability such as when prolonged sustained activity depletes glycogen stores. It is doubtful that this occurs in any of the common competitive events but it is likely to be an issue during routine intense training and during prolonged marathon swimming.

The neuromuscular junction has also been implicated as a potential source of fatigue. We have already described how fatigue can be mediated by transmitter depletion within theCNS. Other research has shown that depletion of transmitters at the end of motor neurons can also result in decreases in muscular force. Clearly, the causes of fatigue are varied and are a function of the intensity of the exercise bout, its duration, the physiological traits of the athlete, and the athlete's training state. Different athletes might fatigue for different reasons even when participating in a similar swim workout. The important point here is that the CNS is likely an important contributor to strength and power as well as fatigue. During the training plan, careful consideration must be given to the specific effects training might have on CNS function.

Muscle fiber type

The specific traits of the muscle fibers are thought to be, in part, dictated by the nerve fibers that innervate them. They can be differentiated as well by the characteristics of the proteins involved in the fiber's contractile apparatus (Fig. 3.3). Fibers that have high myofibriller ATPase activity also have high maximum velocities of shortening and are thus referred to as "fast twitch." Slow-twitch fibers have low ATPase activity and take longer to reach peak tension. Muscles in the body are generally composed of different percentages of slow and fast-twitch fibers seemingly reflected by how these muscles are used.

A motor unit, the motor neuron and all of the fibers that are innervated by it, is the fundamental functional unit of muscular activity. The metabolic characteristics of the fibers within a given motor unit can also be defined. Typically one of the mitochondrial enzymes involved in oxidative metabolism is qualitatively assessed. This results in assigning either high or low activity to oxidative characteristics of the fiber. This has led to classification of muscle fibers as being Type I or II, slow or fast. In addition, the oxidative capacity of fast-twitch fibers can be classified as high oxidative (IIa) or low oxidative (IIb). Several additional fiber types have been described, with the most notable of these being Type IIx. This latter fiber type has been suggested to be somewhere between IIa and IIb as far

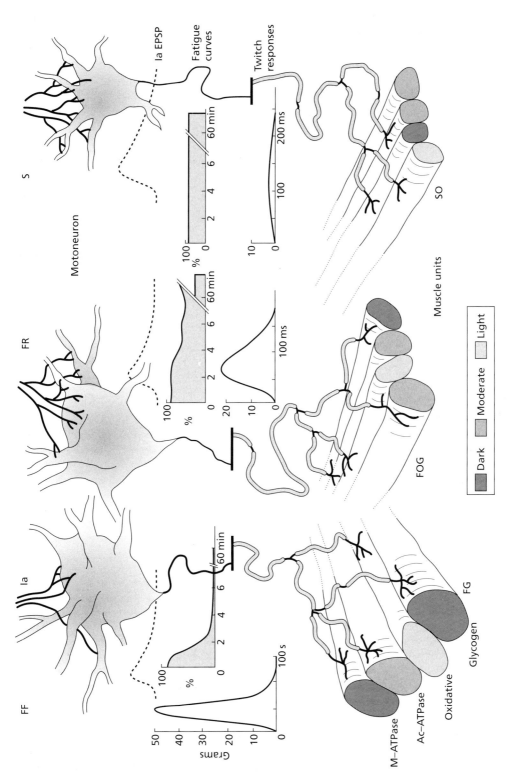

Fig. 3.3 Fundamental properties of the fast-contracting fatigable (FF), fast-contracting fatigue-resistant (FR), and slow-contracting fatigue-resistant (S) motor units in relation to recruitment order, tension development, fatigue resistance, myosin adenosine triphosphatase activity, oxidative capacity, and glycogen content. FG, fast glycolytic; FOG, fast oxidative glycolytic; SO, slow oxidative; 1a, nerve; EPSP, excitatory postsynaptic potential. Reproduced with permission from *Skeletal Muscle Structure and Function: Implications for Rehabilitation and Sports Medicine* (ed. R.L. Lieber), 1992, Lippincott Williams & Wilkins, Philadelphia, PA.

as power is concerned, but similar to IIa metabolically. Recently described differences in the myosin protein have led researchers to suggest that muscle fibers may some day be further subdivided into many distinct subcategories.

These specific traits act to influence the motor unit's tendency to fatigue. The important point here is recognizing that the fast-twitch fibers contribute more force at high limb speeds than do the slow-twitch fibers. Postural muscles, which are fatigue-resistant, are largely slow twitch, while the prime movers have a greater proportion of fast-twitch fibers.

While certain biochemical traits can be shifted through training, most of the evidence suggests that muscle fiber type is largely influenced by the CNS and heredity. The significance of this is self-evident and supports the contention that sprinters might indeed be born, rather than developed. So too is the suggestion that by attempting to improve a sprinter's endurance capacity it is just as likely that you will compromise their sprint performance as improve it.

Force–velocity relationship

Other factors specifically related to the architecture of the muscle also affect muscular strength and power. As noted earlier, the rate at which the muscle myofibrils shorten is a function of the inherent enzymatic makeup of the fiber and is used as a means of differentiating one fiber type from another. Fiber-shortening velocity is an important factor in determining muscle force output that makes the relationship between strength and power even more complicated (Fig. 3.4). When a muscle fiber is stimulated to contract, the rate at which it does so is affected by the tension it is required to develop. The greater the tension or resistance the muscle must overcome, the slower the velocity of shortening. When a fiber is required to shorten with little or no resistance, the velocity of shortening is very high and power is high as well. At the maximal force that a fiber can generate, there is no shortening and thus the power falls to zero. The relationship between force and velocity dictates that the maximal power a fiber can generate occurs when the fiber exerts about one third of its maximal tension. It has been suggested that changes in power following a training program are most evident at the velocity at which the muscle is trained. Training at a slow velocity

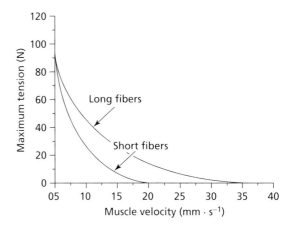

Fig. 3.4 Length–tension and force–velocity plots for muscles with identical cross-sectional areas but short and long fiber lengths. From *Skeletal Muscle Structure, Function, and Plasticity* (ed. R.L. Lieber), 2nd edn, p. 73, 1997, Lippincott Williams & Wilkins, Philadelphia, PA, with permission.

might improve strength without much effect at the faster shortening velocities typically observed during swimming.

Added to this relationship is the observation that the rate at which a muscle shortens is related to its length. Longer muscles shorten faster at a given tension than short muscles because of the fact that there are more muscle contractile "units" in series in the longer fibers (Fig. 3.4). These characteristics may prove to be important in terms of conferring success in the various swim events.

Skeletal muscle mass

Athletes have little control over many of these factors but because of the importance of power as a determinant of maximum swim velocity, specific power training is almost universally included as a critical component of a swimmer's training program. This should be included if for no other reason than to increase the muscle mass (and cross-sectional area) of the prime movers. Invoking specific changes in muscle mass through the swim season, however, has proven difficult for the typical swim coach. As it turns out, muscle mass changes have also been difficult for the physiologist to measure.

For the purpose of body composition analysis, it is often common for researchers to use a two-compartment model. The two compartments generally assessed are the fat compartment, which is composed of primarily fat storage tissues, and the lean compartment, which is composed of skeletal muscle, bone, and the internal organs. While fat mass has only a nominal association with swim performance, the relationship between lean body mass and performance in swimming is clear. Thus, of specific interest to us is quantification of the portion of the lean mass that is composed primarily of skeletal muscle mass. Unfortunately, a simple direct measure of muscle mass has proven to be nearly impossible to identify.

In an average individual the skeletal muscle mass represents nearly two thirds of the lean mass, or approximately 40 kg. Nearly 75% of this muscle weight is water. In the laboratory, the water can be removed from a muscle sample through dehydration. Most of what remains of the muscle is composed of contractile protein. While the weight of the remaining protein is not impressive (less than 15 kg of total body weight), it is this protein that accounts for most of the physiological work done during exercise, i.e., the mechanical power produced. Newer, expensive techniques such as magnetic resonance imaging (MRI) and nuclear magnetic resonance (NMR) allow quantification of muscle mass by looking at discrete cross-sectional images. Because of the expense (approximately $1000 per image), however, these techniques will be of limited use to the average swim coach (Fig. 3.5).

One field measure that does allow an estimate of the muscle mass, at least of the upper arm, can be obtained by using skinfold calipers and a tape measure. Fat mass, as estimated by the skinfold thickness, is subtracted from cross-sectional area to derive an estimate of mid-upper arm cross-sectional muscle area (CSMA). The equation for CSMA is

$$CSMA = (MUAC - \pi\,TricepSF)^2 / 4\pi$$

where MUAC is mid-upper arm circumference and TricepSF is triceps skinfold. We have used this measure in our research and have shown it to be highly related to sprint swim performance. Mean CSMA for female swimmers was 42 cm^2 ($N = 132$) while mean area for males was 62 cm^2 ($N = 127$).

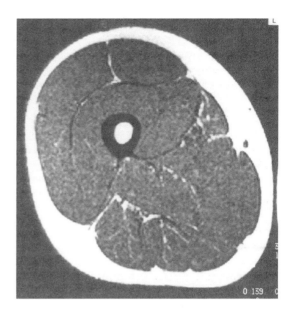

Fig. 3.5 Cross section of the thigh obtained by MRI. Muscle, fat, and bone components are clearly visible.

Note, however, that strength and power can be influenced by the CNS. In the early stages of training, much of the gain in strength and muscular power output can be attributed to the CNS "learning" to generate more force and power rather than to organic changes (myogenic effects including increased muscle mass) that might occur within the muscle.

Specialization

Specialization in many sports has been suggested to be a function of being on either end of the fiber-type continuum (Table 3.1). Elite sprinters are found to have a high proportion of Type II fibers (perhaps as much as 90%) in the muscles responsible for acceleration of the limbs. Distance athletes are reported to have a high distribution of Type I fibers. Keep in mind that a muscle can contain a mixture of fiber types, with some muscles consisting predominantly of Type I fibers while other muscles are mostly Type II. For example, postural muscles tend to be predominantly Type I while muscles of the limbs tend to have a greater percentage of Type II fibers.

Table 3.1 The average percentage of slow-twitch (%ST) and fast-twitch (%FT) fibers in selected muscles of male (M) and female (F) athletes. (Also shown are the average cross-sectional areas of the muscle fibers.) From *Swimming* (D.L. Costill, E.W. Maglischo & A.B. Richardson), 1st edn, p. 6, 1992, Blackwell Science Ltd, Oxford, UK.

Athletes	Sex	Muscle	%ST	%FT	Fiber size (μ^2)	
					ST	FT
Swimmers	M	Deltoidius	67	33	6345	5455
	F	Deltoidius	69	31	4332	3857
Sprint (runners)	M	Gastrocnemius	24	76	5878	6034
	F	Gastrocnemius	27	73	3752	3930
Distance (runners)	M	Gastrocnemius	79	21	8342	6485
	F	Gastrocnemius	69	31	4441	4128
Cyclists	M	Vastus lateralis	57	43	6333	6116
	F	Vastus lateralis	51	49	5487	5216
Weightlifters	M	Gastrocnemius	44	56	5060	8910
	M	Deltoidius	53	47	5010	8450
Triathletes	M	Deltoidius	60	40	–	–
	M	Vastus lateralis	63	37	–	–
	M	Gastrocnemius	59	41	–	–
Canoeists	M	Deltoidius	71	29	4920	7040
Shot-putters	M	Gastrocnemius	38	62	6367	6441
Nonathletes	M	Vastus lateralis	47	53	4722	4709

The difficulty for coaches who are training swimmers is that extensive, prolonged, exhaustive swim practices tend to present cellular and central changes consistent with improved muscular endurance rather than improved muscular power. In other words, it has been shown to be difficult to improve both the capacity to generate high muscular power outputs and the capacity to improve muscular endurance simultaneously. This is true even though the limiting factors for the two traits are different. The type of training that influences one cellular trait in a positive manner seems to compromise the other.

A relevant question is: does a typical age group swim training program favor sprinters or endurance athletes? The answer to this question is dependent upon the unique training plan of the swimmer's coach. It is tempting to hypothesize that individuals with a mixed muscle fiber type might hold an advantage at younger ages until the expression of other inherent traits is fully realized. However, while muscular endurance can be enhanced in young children, the ability to increase aerobic capacity is limited until the middle teens. Similarly, athletes can increase strength and power through neurological means, but significant gains due to hypertrophic muscular mechanisms only occur postpuberty. The neuroendocrine axis is not mature in young children to the point where phenotypic expression is significantly altered by training until postadolescence. Thus, weight training and power training should probably be postponed until the athletes are physically mature. Or, it should be included in the program at the point where significant gains in muscular power are apparent. The research literature suggests that this might occur at or around the age of 12 or 13 years in girls and 14 or 15 years in boys. This is similar to what has been found to be true for aerobic capacity. Large differences in $\dot{V}o_{2max}$ among athletes become apparent only after puberty, which, on the average, occurs during the early teenage years in both girls and boys. There is not much literature available on the fiber type of young children. Fiber typing is an invasive process that would be difficult to justify for use in children for any purpose.

Sprint muscle

Now we address the prevailing thought on sprinting and sprinters. The muscles involved in moving the limbs of elite sprinters have been shown to contain a high proportion of Type II fibers. In contrast, successful distance athletes are known to have high percentages of Type I fibers in their prime movers. Over the last 25 years, many athletes have been "fiber-typed." The fiber type of the vastus lateralus, for example, varies from athlete to athlete, ranging from nearly 90% fast twitch in elite sprinters to as much as 80 or 90% slow twitch in great distance athletes. An athlete's capacity to sustain high-intensity work can be dependent upon the distribution of the fibers within the muscle cells. Fiber type may influence their "trainability" as well as their ultimate potential to excel in the various events and distances.

Because the Type IIb fibers are highly fatigable, these fibers tend to be recruited only when absolutely necessary. Thus it is thought that coaches must fatigue the swimmers' Type IIa and I fibers before training will have any appreciable effect upon the Type IIb fibers. For this reason, many coaches plan their workouts, with intensity and power output increasing as the swim practice continues. In other words, coaches decrease the interval distance and increase the rest interval as practice progresses in an attempt to recruit and load the Type II fibers as the Type I fibers gradually fatigue. An alternate approach, that may be equally, if not more, valid, is to simply allow the sprinters to swim fast prior to onset of significant general muscular fatigue (Fig. 3.6). When maximal power is required, the CNS learns to recruit the Type II fibers quicker. For the sprinter, success lies in the ability of the skeletal muscle to generate force (strength) quickly (power) and the ability to apply it efficiently (stroke technique) to the water. Sprinters rely on immediate phosphogen energy sources and glycolysis and only secondarily upon factors consistent with the aerobic pathways and

endurance. Sprinters are less reliant on central adaptations, cardiac and pulmonary responses, as compared to the distance athlete. Distance athletes, in contrast, are able to endure partially because of peripheral muscular enzymatic adaptations (peripheral endurance) and partially because of robust cardiorespiratory capacities (central endurance). The distance athlete excels as a function of the adaptive structural and functional responses of the heart, lung, and blood, peripheral vascular changes, as well as several very specific peripheral skeletal muscle adaptations.

Because the skeletal muscles comprise nearly 50% of body weight, they represent the major site of metabolic activity at rest and during exercise. Their select traits largely determine an individual's capacity to adapt to training and success in the various swim events. While virtually any competitive swimmer can complete a 1500-m swim, only truly elite men can complete the swim in 15 min or less. Similarly, many swimmers can finish a 100-m swim in under a minute. Only a few men can swim it in under 50 s. Optimal, specific swim training and favorable genetics combine to allow exceptional performances of this nature.

However, the effect of much of conventional swim training seems to be beneficial for enhancing the endurance capacity of the athlete without altering his or her ability to sprint. This pattern of training encourages cardiopulmonary adaptations and enhances the endurance traits of both Type I and II fibers without enhancing muscular power output. To emphasize these points, the next sections will focus on the specifics of the sprinter and the distance swimmer separately.

The sprinter

The importance of good sprint performance is evident in team competitions in swimming, as not only are there many points scored from multiple short individual events, but sprinters contribute vitally important relay points. Despite the old adage "when the going gets tough, the sprinters get out," champion sprint swimmers train extensively and successful coaches must necessarily be successful sprint coaches. In a program to optimally develop sprinters it is not uncommon to find sprinters practicing long after the distance swimmers have finished. Counsilman, the swim

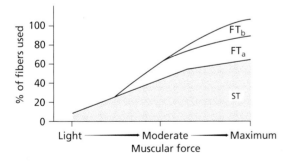

Fig. 3.6 The ramp-like recruitment of muscle fibers with varied levels of muscular effort. While light force requirements only use the slow-twitch fibers, heavy loads on the muscle will result in the recruitment of all three types of muscle fibers. From *Swimming* (D.L. Costill, E.W. Maglischo & A.B. Richardson), 1st edn, p. 5, 1992, Blackwell Science Ltd, Oxford, UK.

coach at Indiana University noted for training innovation, instituted a program for his swimmers that frequently required three practices a day. The third practice became known as Sprinter's Delight and resulted in many national and international record sprint performances.

As noted earlier, there has always been debate as to how to correctly train a sprinter and what that training should entail. Some coaches have been heard to conclude that sprinters are born or *recruited*, while distance swimmers are *developed*. We have already established that to some extent, for truly exceptional performers, both sprinters and endurance swimmers are genetically gifted and optimally trained. Nevertheless, it has been many years since any swimmer, sprint or otherwise, has been successful at the elite level without an extensive training regimen.

Physical characteristics

Coaches often refer to certain individuals as "pure sprinters" or "drop dead" sprinters. The pure sprinter is an athlete that has difficulty performing at a high level throughout a practice session, let alone throughout a week of multiple practices per day. These individuals appear to be able to sprint for 20–30 s (swim the 50 or 100 m) and fatigue at distances less than 100 m. While this is an empirical observation from the coach's perspective, not much research has been focused specifically on "sprint-like" activity. The reason for this is simple. Sprint activity cannot be sustained beyond a fraction of a minute and thus careful analysis of the physiologic and cellular determinants of sprinting is nearly impossible. Time, or in this case the lack of time, is the culprit.

Are there ways of assessing the "explosiveness" of a swimmer without invasive muscle biopsy procedures? Studies suggest that dryland measures that are somewhat useful include the standing vertical jump and the two-hand chest pass. More sensitive measures are those obtained in the water and include measuring power via the use of a pulley-weight system such as the commercially available Power Rack®. The procedure involves having the athlete swim against progressively increasing resistance while recording their time and stroke count. Maximal power and power per stroke can be measured in this manner and accounts for nearly 90% of the variance in maximal swim velocity.

Approaches available to describe other determinants of sprint swimming include using a cross-sectional sample of a diverse population of sprinters. Another approach is to try to understand the underlying fluid dynamic principles that contribute to maximal swim velocity. This will be the primary focus of Chapters 4 and 5. Swimming fast is a balance between propulsive forces and resistive forces. The relationship between propulsive and resistive forces is such that resistive forces are largely represented by the water and increase with the square of the swimmer's velocity. Thus, as the velocity of the swimmer increases, the muscular power required to swim just a bit faster increases at an ever-greater rate, proportional to the increase in resistance. Swimming fast, at velocities at or above $2 \text{ m} \cdot \text{s}^{-1}$, requires a tremendous generation of muscular force, an ability to generate it quickly, and the ability to apply the force efficiently and effectively. It would appear that the power output required to achieve this velocity is such that metabolically it is very difficult to sustain for much more than a minute. Nevertheless, the sprinter's skeletal muscles (and perhaps the sprinter's other specific anthropometric and physiologic characteristics) play a large role in this regard. Therefore, the two components of speed in swimming are those inherent traits that convey muscular *and* mechanical power and the neuromotor traits that determine technique or skill.

Clearly the relationship between strength, power, and swim velocity is complicated to a large extent by those traits that dictate technique, or rather the mechanical application of the strength and power to the water, resulting in forward motion. The traits that favor the generation of mechanical power include height and arm length. Prominent sprinters tend to be taller than average height. Arm span (from finger tip to finger tip with the arms perpendicular to the body) is generally equal to body height. In talented sprinters, arm span tends to be 6–10% greater than height. Hand size is important, as is foot size. Surprisingly, the best sprinters are also shown to be the best kickers, and maximal kick velocity correlates with sprint swim time very highly.

While having a high Type IIb component is beneficial, in terms of explosiveness and maximal power output, the down side of this is that the traits that favor fatigue resistance are greatly absent. In line with symmorphosis, the capacities of the various systems seem to be in balance with the demand placed upon them. Capillary density is low in muscles with a high percentage of Type IIb. Mitochondrial mass is low. Myoglobin content is low. The enzymes needed for maintaining high rates of aerobic metabolism are likewise lower than that found in slow-twitch fibers. When recruited to produce force, these muscles are supplied energy by the pathways that do not require oxygen. As a result, however, from a metabolic perspective, they are unable to endure.

Training

One problem in terms of training the sprinter is that the adaptability of the Type II fibers is low as far as metabolic pathways are concerned. These fibers do appear to be able to respond to simultaneous sprint and endurance training. Hypertrophy does occur with strength training, with an increase in myofibriller content. Force production and power output increase proportionately. Enzymes, mostly glycolytic enzymes, responsible for generating energy from the available substrates, however, are only likely to increase by 10–15% with sprint training. Immediate energy supplies increase little or only proportional to the increase in muscle mass. This contrasts to the 200–300% increase in the aerobic enzyme concentrations in the slow-twitch fiber with endurance training. What appears to occur then is when the fast-twitch fibers increase their ability to generate force and power to a significant degree with appropriate training, the ability to supply the energy required to sustain this power is only marginally increased. The "holy grail" of sprint coaching is referred to as "sprint-specific endurance." Coaches are looking for training tactics that will increase maximal power output and help to sustain it for as long as possible.

On the metabolic basis alone, the prediction might be that improvements in short sprint performance come from strength gains and sprint training, leading to greater instantaneous power output with little or no increase (and maybe even a decrease) in the ability to resist fatigue. An example might be that over 100 m, the athlete with a preponderance of Type II fibers can be trained to take it out faster but the drop-off between the first and second halves might remain approximately the same. The improvements in short sprint performance comes primarily in the first half

of the race, rather than relative improvements in the second half. For the "pure sprinter," the only tactic available might be to train the front end of the race and "get out fast," as the ability to bring it back might be inherent and of limited trainability.

As a coach, it is tempting to attempt to establish a significant aerobic base by interval or over-distance training with short rest. The problem lies in the fact that if you overtrain a sprinter using programs that enhance fatigue resistance and stimulate aerobic metabolism, more likely than not, the sprinter's ability to sprint will not be enhanced, rather only compromised. The specificity of training applies at the cellular level as well as to the whole body. Sprinters who undergo extensive over-distance training and training to improve aerobic capacity generally express a decrease in their explosive power output. It is nearly impossible to train for explosiveness and endurance at the same time without compromising the traits that lead to explosiveness.

It is important to remember that much of the improved power output gained by sprint swimmers is neurological rather than biochemical. There is scientific evidence that shows endurance training might reduce the excitability of the motor neurons. This can be interpreted as reducing the recruitment of muscle fibers given the same central motor stimulus. Mid-season declines in explosiveness might be of CNS origin rather than peripheral or muscular as is generally assumed.

When a sprinter is trained using a program designed to increase endurance, many changes are evident. As might be expected, mitochondrial volume is increased and subsequently there is an improvement in aerobic enzyme concentration. While this improves the swimmers' ability to sustain submaximal swim velocities and their ability to recover from intensive bouts of exercise, their ability to sprint is significantly deteriorated. The Type IIb fibers lose cross-sectional area and the ability to produce power through non-robic means is also reduced. With an increased mitochondrial volume comes the increased ability to "clear" lactate evidenced by lower blood lactate values and a shift in OBLA. This would act to favor a quicker recovery but not necessarily improve performance *per se*.

Consistent with Noakes' revised model of fatigue, sprinters may need to "recover" from training, while the distance swimmer only needs to rest. This is in line with the observation that swim times only improve after the sprint athlete is fully recovered and tapered. The distance swimmer might show continued improvement as systemic and enzymatic adaptations continue to occur. The question therefore becomes: is continued aerobic training optimal or even necessary for the sprinter? Some coaches today believe that sprinters can train hard and swim well year-round without approaching the point of general exhaustion or becoming overtrained.

An interesting observation that might be of relevance here is the possibility that muscle fibers might also self-regulate specific traits as a function of their metabolic needs. When high rates of aerobic metabolism are required, the muscle fiber may limit hypertrophy specifically as a means to achieve optimal diffusion of respiratory gases into and out of the cell. Diffusion is, in part, related to the distance or tissue thickness across which the gases diffuse. Thus, the maximal diffusion rates within muscle tissues are a function of the distances between the capillary and the intracellular mitochondrial matrix. Increases in the aerobic capacity of the muscle at some point will require increased capillary density and increased mitochondrial mass per volume of muscle tissue. These increases must be proportional to any gains in muscle mass, and may be greater. This assumes, of course, that the various components of the system are roughly matched and that symmorphosis drives function.

What this says in simple terms is that distance swimmers and ultra-marathoners cannot afford the relative muscularity of the sprint swimmer when viewed from a cellular metabolic basis alone. It may be that the need for high diffusion rates acts to limit the amount of muscle hypertrophy that can be sustained maximally. On the other hand, sprinters who are limited in their performances by the ability to generate muscular power may not necessarily be helped in these short events by improving their aerobic potential. In the world of the sprinter, the goal is strictly to increase instantaneous power output while minimizing the various elements of resistance.

Sprint talent identification

Is it possible that competitive swim programs "weed out" pure sprinters by the time they reach high school?

This seems to be a distinct possibility even though, in the United States at least, much of the competition for the younger age groups tends to be short sprint-type events. Despite this, many coaches seem to be training their young athletes to endure the practice sessions rather than to be able to swim specific competitive events. The pure sprinter may be successful in meets when adequately rested but may have difficulty practicing with any sustained quality. Alternatively, once swimmers reach their middle teens, many of the purely sprint events are eliminated from age group competitions and emphasis is placed more upon middle distance events. Practice distances and practice expectations rise such that the sprinter can easily become discouraged and eventually quit. While it is common practice at the collegiate level to identify a sprint group and train them accordingly, few age group coaches have the time or personnel to be able to do so. Furthermore, the expression of the underlying inherited traits, the phenotype of an individual, becomes more apparent postpuberty.

General conclusions on sprinters

With this information in mind, if a perfect sprinter could be designed, what would one look like? Muscularity would be a great trait to start with though not all sprinters exactly fit the stereotype. Tall, large hands, broad shoulders, long arms and legs, lean, muscular with big feet would be included in a set of traits that might define our perfect sprinter. Interestingly, these are virtually the same traits that Johnny Weissmuller (who in the 1920s once held every sprint freestyle world record) listed nearly 70 years ago when asked to describe what made him a great sprinter. One need only look toward Gary Hall Jr., Alexander Popov, Matt Biondi, Pieter van den Hoogenband, Jim Montgomery, and others to see that similar traits remain appropriate today. However, this does not mean that these specific traits are absolute requirements for outstanding sprint performance, as there are always successful individuals who might be seen as exceptions to these generalities. In these cases, it may be the intangible factors that contribute the most to outstanding performance. The sport psychologist might be right in stating that winning is 90% mental and 10% physical.

Distance swimmers

The elite distance athlete is much tougher to describe. To a greater extent the ability to excel at the longer competitive events is much less dictated by anthropometric traits (height, arm span, etc.) than are the sprint events. This may be due to the importance of the "distance swimmer's mentality," or to less apparent physiological characteristics.

As the event distance increases, the contribution of the aerobic pathway to performance increases. As such, the importance of the match between mitochondrial respiration and the ability to supply the tissues with necessary metabolic substrates become paramount. Unfortunately, there are few external clues to an individual's mitochondrial mass. Cardiac volumes are also impossible to casually assess. Performance-related variables must therefore be used by coaches to predict endurance talent.

Physiologists are confident that the rate at which food energy can be converted to physiologically available energy largely determines swim performance. In distance events, this conversion rate is primarily a function of mitochondrial respiration and the ability of the cardiorespiratory system to supply the peripheral tissues with substrates. These are reflected in the assessment of aerobic capacity ($\dot{V}_{O2max}$) and the anaerobic threshold.

The difficulty in assessing these values in swimmers is that the most accurate means of doing so requires that it be done while swimming. Because of the need for ventilatory volumes and expired gas analysis, measuring the $\dot{V}_{O2max}$ in swimmers is far from routine. The development of swim flumes has eased the problems and yet the accessibility to the few flumes in existence has limited the value to coaches. It should also be recognized that the ability to significantly alter $\dot{V}_{O2max}$ through training is only apparent after puberty. Research has shown that children express a surprisingly similar aerobic capacity up to the early teenage years irrespective of their sex. This may be one explanation for why girls can compete with boys on an even basis until this age.

In contrast to the very high values obtained from elite cross-country skiers (in excess of 80 ml $O_2 \cdot kg^{-1} \cdot min^{-1}$), $\dot{V}_{O2max}$ values for swimmers are much lower (on the order of 55–65 ml $\cdot kg^{-1} \cdot min^{-1}$).

There are potentially two reasons for these findings. First, it is known that $\dot{V}_{O2max}$ is a function of the muscle mass being employed during the exercise. Swimming uses the muscles of the chest, arms, and back, and secondarily the trunk, and leg muscles. It is suggested that the muscle mass employed during swimming is thus less than perhaps cycling or running. Secondly, when the values for swimmers are reported, they are not commonly separated by event. Thus, the values for sprinters, mid-distance, and distance swimmers are pooled, or averaged, and only a single value is reported. It is likely that the distance athletes have significantly higher values for $\dot{V}_{O2max}$ when compared to the sprinters, similar to what is reported for athletes in other sports.

The anaerobic threshold was originally proposed as the point whereby oxygen became limited during a progressive test. We now know that except during near-maximal or maximal exercise, oxygen consumption does not appear limited by oxygen availability. The threshold, as indexed by the appearance of lactic acid levels in the blood and nonlinear increases in ventilation, is now seen as a marker of balance between aerobic and non-oxygen-consuming metabolic pathways. As such, it is a better predictor of success in endurance events than is $\dot{V}_{O2max}$. The optimal combination for outstanding performance is a high $\dot{V}_{O2max}$ and a high anaerobic threshold. The high $\dot{V}_{O2max}$ comes as a result of a high mitochondrial metabolic capacity and the cardiovascular capacity to deliver oxygen and other necessary substrates at a rapid rate. Peripheral tissue adaptations include high tissue vascularity, high mitochondrial volumes, high myoglobin concentrations, and enzymatic adaptations allowing high rates of fat metabolism.

It is possible to train an athlete who might be a genotypic sprinter to express a distance athlete's phenotype. Aerobic training tends to "push" the inherent fiber type toward the metabolic traits of the Type I fiber. The neurological traits of the fiber are fixed, yet the metabolic variables can shift toward the endurance end. Changes in the properties of the contractile proteins are also a real possibility.

There is nothing to suppose that the hydrodynamics of propulsion and resistance in human swimming are different between sprint and endurance events. However, because of the relationship that exists between drag and swim velocity, technique may be more of an issue in distance swimming than it is in sprint swimming.

Distance events

The pure distance events are the 800- and 1500-m freestyles. Although the 400 freestyle and 400 individual medley may be considered by some to be distance events, they are more properly classified as middle-distance, but usually serve as companions to the longer swims. Relative to running, Olympic swimming has no true distance event comparable to the marathon. The energy systems used during 400-, 800-, 1500-m races lasting approximately 4, 8, and 16 min, respectively, compare more favorably to running distances between 1500 m and 5 km than the energy systems used during the marathon. Unlike running, it is common to see distance swimmers compete in all the events, from 50 to 1500 m, at some point in a season. For example, a distance swimmer may be required to swim a fast 200 on a relay. Hence, the distance swimmer uses all the energy systems and types of training discussed in this book, but in different proportions than the sprint swimmer.

Physical characteristics

A picture of the typical distance swimmer and distance training over the past 30 years can be constructed from opinions expressed by successful distance coaches at the American Swimming Coaches Association World Clinics (Distance Training School, 1997).

Distance swimmers come in all shapes and sizes, but just as the distance runner must have a high strength-to-weight ratio, so must the distance swimmer. The characteristics discussed previously that infer high aerobic capacity are essential—high mitochondrial density, high percent of slow-twitch fibers, large cardiac output, etc. Some of the best distance swimmers have been tall, slender, buoyant, flexible, light-framed, and lightly muscled, i.e., they look like distance runners. Because of their fiber type, they usually are not good jumpers.

Endurance ability is evident at an early age. The budding distance swimmer may not be the fastest member of the team, but can sustain a high energy output for

a long time and can withstand more training volume than the rest of the team. At the elite level, the most successful distance swimmers tend to be younger than the most successful sprinters. For example, over the past decade at the US Long Course Nationals, the average age of the women finalists in the 1500 m was 16.8 years, compared to 21.3 years for the finalists in the 50-m freestyle. The men show a similar pattern. The average age of the finalists in the men's 1500 m was 19.8 years compared to 23.4 years for the finalists in the 50-m freestyle.

Mental characteristics

It takes a certain type of person to be a distance swimmer, one with the attitude and work ethic necessary to enjoy performing difficult workouts day in and day out, even doing more than is required. Distance swimmers enjoy hard work and competition, both in practice and at meets. They enjoy competing against the clock and have a keen sense of pace. Distance swimming requires concentration, and it has been said that smart people win the distance events, especially long course meters. Distance swimmers have an awareness of what they are doing in practice and want to know why they are doing it. Other common descriptors for the personality of the distance swimmer include easy-going, low key, well organized, independent, doers, and well adapted.

Training

It takes careful preparation to succeed as a distance swimmer. As Bill Sweetenham says, "The best prepared swimmers win the 1500." Although the volume of training performed by distance swimmers has fluctuated over the past several decades, it is universally accepted that in order to be successful, one must work very hard, not only in terms of volume of work, but quality as well. The typical volume seems to be about 80 000 m per week in 10–11 workouts, with some anaerobic work for speed. There is no secret, just lots of hard work. Dick Jochums summarizes distance training as follows: "The key for the distance swimmer is to get as much short rest work at race pace as possible." It is important to maintain consistent, high mileage, high-quality training. Being a distance swimmer is a full-time job, so it's dangerous to take too much time off between seasons.

Good technique is essential, as is an awareness of pace learned through negative split and descend sets in practice. The goal is to swim the race in practice, using the same even splits used in a meet. A long, challenging set or timed swim once a week is recommended. Many distance coaches also prescribe more pulling drills for their distance swimmers. Some coaches do no dryland strength training with their distance swimmers, preferring to gain strength in the water through pulling drills, while others have their swimmers perform body weight exercises, or light weight/high repetition strength training, 3 days a week.

Although some young swimmers enjoy the distance events because improvement is rapid, the increase in training volume and intensity should be developed slowly over years, with an emphasis on aerobic work at a young age. It may not be wise to start two-a-day sessions before puberty.

Taper

Because distance events are physically and emotionally demanding, it is not wise to race the long events too often. The length of the taper depends on age, muscle mass, length of the race, and the mental characteristics of the athlete. Older and more heavily muscled swimmers usually need a longer taper. Longer races usually require less taper. Some distance swimmers do not respond well to a taper, mentally or physically, and perform better with very little rest. Experience is the best teacher. No more than two tapers per year should be scheduled, each lasting from 10 days to 3 weeks. Double workouts can be maintained but strength training should be discontinued 3 weeks before the big meet. Men may need up to 3 weeks of taper, with a decrease in intensity during the first week, followed by a drop in distance the last 2 weeks, and nothing too hard the last 10 days. Women may respond better to less taper, perhaps only 8–10 days total. Despite these recommendations, each athlete should be treated as an individual and should not be forced to do hard efforts during the taper if they do not feel well. It is a time to prepare psychologically for the big meet, with an emphasis on broken swims at race pace to build confidence. Dick Jochums sums up the taper phase in

one sentence: "The taper, for the distance freestyler, is basically a two-week period of race rehearsal and rest."

Motivation

The key to a successful distance program is a close relationship between the swimmer and the coach, because it is the coach who creates an attitude and an environment that promotes hard work. "The way to make it fun is to create enthusiasm for the event, highlight the event, prioritize the event and put distance swimmers together as frequently as possible to train, not to compete. They will compete by simple training together" (Bill Sweetenham). "In my mind, there is no secret when it comes to endurance training. The key is that the coach must motivate the athlete to train hard on a consistent basis" (Mark Schubert).

Conclusions

The proteins within the skeletal muscles comprise the microfilaments that generate force. To generate force, however, requires metabolic support via energy production within the cells. This must be accompanied by cardiovascular changes and the ability to supply the muscles with needed substrates. Skeletal muscle adaptations and secondary central adaptations that support the specific muscular adaptations must be a primary focus of swim coaches whose job it is to improve the athlete's performance through daily training. It is therefore important to have a sophisticated understanding of skeletal muscle function and how training may alter the muscle's (and the athlete's) capacity to do work and resist fatigue.

There seems to be a dichotomy between adaptations that result in power and those that promote endurance such that it is difficult to enhance both at once. Workouts that exhaust an athlete who has predominantly fast-twitch Type II fibers might only marginally challenge the athlete who has predominantly Type I prime movers.

So, to answer the question that was posed in the introduction to this chapter: Are successful sprinters inherently different from successful endurance swimmers, or is it more a matter of training? The answer is: Yes! Elite sprinters are different from elite distance swimmers. In addition, they train differently to enhance those traits necessary for success in their respective events. Central factors as well as important metabolic and inherent peripheral traits characterize individuals and tend to favor success in specific events. Because of the unique combination of requirements necessary for success, training must be specific and strategies for training swimmers must be founded upon each individual's inherent traits.

Recommended reading

ASCA (1997) *Distance Training School. A Collection of Presentations Given at the ASCA World Clinic 1972–1995.* Ft Lauderdale, FL: American Swimming Coaches Association.

Barany, M. (1967) ATPase activity of myosin correlated with speed of muscle shortening. *Journal of General Physiology* **50**, 197–216.

Bergstrom, J. (1967) Local changes of ATP and phosphocreatine in human muscle tissue in connection with exercise. *Circulation Research* **21**, 191–198.

Bigland-Ritchie, B., Johnson, R., Lippold, O. & Woods, J.J. (1983) Contractile speed and EMG changes during fatigue of sustained maximal voluntary contractions. *Journal of Neurophysiology* **50**, 313–324.

Buller, A.J., Eccles, J.C. & Eccles, R.M. (1960) Interactions between motorneurons and muscles in respect to the characteristic speeds of their responses. *Journal of Physiology (London)* **150**, 417–439.

Costill, D.L., Rayfield, F., Kirwan, J. & Thomas, R. (1986) A computer based system for the measurement of force and power during front crawl swimming. *Journal of Swimming Research* **2**, 16–19.

Edstrom, L. & Kugelberg, E. (1968) Histochemical composition distribution of fibers and fatigability of single motor units. *Journal of Neurology, Neurosurgery and Psychiatry* **31**, 424–433.

Eisenberg, B.R. (1983) Quantitative ultrastructure of mammalian skeletal muscle. In: L.D. Peachey, R.H. Adrian & S.R. Geiger, eds. *Skeletal Muscle, Vol. 10.* Baltimore, MD: American Physiological Society, pp. 73–112.

Fukunaga, T., Roy, R.R., Shellock, F.G., Hodgon, J.A., Day, M.K., Lee, P.L., Kwong, F.H. & Edgerton, V.R. (1992) Physiological cross sectional area of human leg muscle based upon magnetic resonance imaging. *Journal of Orthopedic Research* **10**, 928–934.

Henneman, E., Somjen, G. & Carpenter, D.O. (1965) Functional significance of cell size in spinal motorneurons. *Journal of Neurophysiology* **28**, 560–580.

Hill, A.V. (1970) *First and Last Experiments in Muscle Mechanics.* New York: Cambridge University Press.

Holmer, I. (1972) Oxygen uptake during swimming in man. *Journal of Applied Physiology* **33**, 502–509.

Holmer, I. (1974) Physiology of swimming man. *Acta Physiologica Scandinavica* **407**(Suppl.), 1–55.

Podolsky, R.J. & Shoenberg, M. (1983) Force generation and shortening in skeletal muscle. In: *Handbook of Physiology, Vol. 10.* Baltimore, MD: American Physiological Society, pp. 173–187.

Rohrs, D.M. & Stager, J.M. (1991) Evaluation of anaerobic power and capacity in competitive swimmers. *Journal of Swimming Research* **7**(3), 12–16.

Saltin, B., Henriksson, J., Nygaard, E., Andersoen, P. & Jansson, E. (1977) Fiber types and metabolic potentials of skeletal muscles in sedentary and endurance runners. *Annals of the New York Academy of Sciences* **301**, 3–29.

Sharp, R.L., Troup, J.P. & Costill, D.L. (1982) Relationship between power and sprint freestyle swimming. *Medicine and Science in Sports and Exercise* **14**, 53–56.

Spudich, J.A. (1994) How molecular motors work. *Nature* **372**, 515–518.

Troup, J.P. (1984) Review: energy systems and training consideration. *Journal of Swimming Research* **1**, 13–16.

Chapter 4
The mechanics of swimming

Barry S. Bixler

Introduction

Mechanics is the field of physics that deals with the laws of motion, and the effects of forces upon objects or the behavior of those objects. Therefore, the mechanics of swimming is the study of how swimmers interact with the water to accomplish motion. The forces behind this motion are highly complex, and an understanding of them requires knowledge of not only the swimmer's motion, but also the motion of the water, and the interaction between the two. That may seem obvious, but in the twentieth century, most swimming scientists, trained in biomechanics but not fluid mechanics, focused mainly on the motion of the swimmer. The motion of the water was usually ignored. However, just as a set of footprints can tell an accomplished tracker many things about a person being tracked (direction, speed, weight, height, etc.), the water motion around and behind a swimmer can reveal many things about the swimmer.

There are sophisticated tools and techniques in use today by engineers and scientists in mainstream engineering fields that can significantly advance the state-of-the-art in swimming mechanics. Most of them remain untapped, however, simply because the swimming community is unaware of them or deems them too complicated. A successful migration of these tools into the field of swimming mechanics would greatly advance the state-of-the-art in swimming. This will, however, require a better understanding of fluid mechanics by the swimming community. The next two chapters contain information designed to assist the reader in acquiring such understanding. Some of the information is standard fare for swimming books, but much of it, derived from the field of fluid mechanics, will be new to the swimming community. With this additional knowledge, it is hoped that swimming scientists will be encouraged to use the more sophisticated tools available to them, and that swim coaches will be provided with useful background information to help them properly interpret and apply the results of such research.

Chapter 4 presents some basic principles of fluid mechanics as they apply to swimming, and by necessity, also contains a number of definitions. Chapter 5 applies the principles presented in Chapter 4 to the two interrelated topics of resistance and propulsion. Although some mathematical equations are shown, the derivations of those equations are not presented, nor do we discuss "how" to perform the four swimming strokes. There are many other books that successfully accomplish those tasks. The goal herein is simple: Show how the principles and concepts of biomechanics and fluid mechanics can be applied to swimming. Many of the examples employed herein to explain these principles involve shapes such as spheres, cylinders, airfoils, etc. These were used because their simple shapes often better demonstrate the principles. More importantly, the research applying these principles to swimmers has not been done.

Some readers may find this material to be too complicated and beyond the requirements of the average swim coach. Consider the following counterpoints to that belief:

• Knowledge will not allow you to be fooled by every newfangled fad that comes along. In the last decade of the twentieth century, science became somewhat unfashionable in some swimming circles, as self-proclaimed gurus preached that neither science nor even hard work made good swimmers. Swimmers had merely to roll their body, or tighten their body, or loosen their body, or they just had to swim like a fish. The scientific basis behind such statements was notably absent, but like the promises of the "elixir" salesmen 100 years ago, their claims were very seductive: Don't think—just pay your money for a seminar and you're home free. As the understanding of the mechanics of swimming increases, such bilking of the swimming community will surely diminish.

• If you understand the swimming research that is underway, you will be able to properly apply the results of such research to develop better swimmers. A scientific approach to stroke design improvement is preferable to the continuation of the trial-and-error method of coaching, which often has coaches jumping from one fad to the next.

• Knowledgeable coaches will help refute the misconception by some outside the swimming community that coaches are coaches because it's the only thing they can do.

• Learn about swimming mechanics because you are a professional who has not lost your enthusiasm for the sport and because you still want to learn everything you can about swimming. When you stop moving forward and do not increase your knowledge, you will stagnate, just like a pool of still water. History is replete with world-renown "experts" who let success go to their head, sat on their laurels, and began to think progress in their fields couldn't possibly go beyond what they themselves knew. Here are a few amusing examples:

Everything that can be invented has been invented. (Charles H. Duell, Director of U.S. Patent Office, 1899)

Who the hell wants to hear actors talk? (Harry M. Warner, Warner Brothers Pictures, c. 1927)

Sensible and responsible women do not want to vote. (Grover Cleveland, 1905)

There is no likelihood man can ever tap the power of the atom. (Robert Millikan, Nobel prize in Physics, 1920)

Ruth made a big mistake when he gave up pitching. (Tris Speaker, 1921)

Heavier than air flying machines are impossible. (Lord Kelvin, President, Royal Society, c. 1895)

Fluid mechanics for swimmers

By necessity, this chapter must include many definitions. Although such lists are as unsavory to the author as they probably are to the readers, they are, unfortunately, a necessary evil. You must first be familiar with the language of fluid mechanics in order to apply it to swimming.

General mechanics definitions

• *Motion* is the process of changing position. Motion may be broken down into two categories: translation and rotation. Translation occurs when all parts of an object travel the same distance in the same direction in the same time. Rotation occurs when all parts of the body rotate about an axis either inside or outside the body, and travel through the same angle and in the same direction in the same time.

• *Speed* is the rate at which an object travels.

• *Velocity* (v) is a speed in a specified direction.

• *Acceleration* (a) is the rate at which velocity changes with time. It may be positive, indicating an increase in velocity with time, or negative, indicating a decrease in velocity with time

• *Acceleration due to gravity* (g) may be taken as a constant 9.8146 m·s^{-2}.

• *Force* (F) is that which produces or tends to produce motion or a change in the motion of bodies. A propulsive force causes motion and a resistive force hinders motion. A force divided by an area equals a pressure.

• *Mass* (m) is the amount of material that an object has, as reflected in its inertia.

• *Weight* (W) is the magnitude of the force of gravity pulling on an object. Mass will always be constant under varying gravitational forces, but weight will change. For example, an astronaut will weigh less on the moon than on the earth, but will have the same mass.

• *Center of gravity* (c.g.) is the point through which the weight of an object appears to act. This is a very important point because it affects a person's balance and stability. For sports applications, the center of gravity of an object is equivalent to the center of mass of an object.

• *Linear momentum* (M) is a quantity of translational motion of a body measured by the product of its mass and velocity. ($M = mV$)

• *Inertia* is a loosely conceived notion that we usually associate with mass. The property of an object that resists setting it in motion or changing its state of motion is its inertia.

• *Moment of inertia* (I) is a property of a body that resists its motion. It is dependent on the mass distribution and the position of the axis of rotation of the body. It is used to determine the angular momentum of a body.

• *Angular velocity* (ω) is the time rate of change of angular rotation about a specified axis.

• *Angular momentum* (L) is a quantity of angular (rotational) motion of a body measured by the product of its moment of inertia and angular velocity. ($L = I\omega$).

Properties and characteristics of a fluid

• *Fluid*—Most common fluids we encounter (such as air and water) may be classified as simple fluids, i.e., they deform continuously when a shear load is applied to them.

• *Density* (ρ) is the mass per unit volume of a substance. The undisturbed mass density of water over the range of environmental conditions encountered by swimmers is essentially a constant (see Table 4.1). However, the swimmer, through stroking and kicking motions, can temporarily modify the water density through the entrainment of air in local areas near the body.

• *Absolute viscosity* (μ) is a property that reveals how much a fluid can resist shearing deformation. It is defined as the shear stress applied to a laminar fluid element divided by the rate of shear strain produced. For example, molasses has a higher viscosity than water.

• *Kinematic viscosity* (ν) is the absolute viscosity divided by the density. It often arises in mathematical treatments of fluid motion. Both the kinematic and absolute viscosity of water change with temperature, another property of water.

• *Compressibility* is a measure of how much a fluid can be compressed. Unless air is entrained in the water, water is essentially incompressible, and as such, is easier to deal with than are compressible fluids such as air.

• *Temperature* (T) is important for swimming fluid mechanics because the viscosity of the water varies with temperature, see Table 4.1.

• *Pressure* (p) is a force per unit area. There exists a pressure at every point within a fluid. When a fluid is flowing around an object, the direction of pressure upon that object is by definition perpendicular to the object's surface. That pressure may be either positive or negative (suction).

• *Hydrostatic pressure* is a pressure that arises in static fluids because any point beneath the surface of a fluid has to support the weight of the fluid above it. The hydrostatic pressure at any point in a fluid is proportional to the depth of that point beneath the free surface.

• *Buoyant force* is a force that is a beneficial consequence of hydrostatic pressure. The upward buoyant force on a body in a fluid is equal to the weight of the fluid displaced by the body. The bottom surface of an object submerged or partially submerged in a fluid has pressure acting on it that is larger than the pressure acting on the top surface of the body. This is because hydrostatic pressure increases with depth of submergence. Thus, the net water force on the body is upward, acting against the force of gravity.

• *Center of buoyancy* is the center of gravity of the water displaced by a body submerged or partially submerged in a fluid.

• *Streamline* is a continuous line drawn through a fluid so that it has the direction of the flow velocity at every point.

• A *fluid particle* is simply a "particle" of fluid that can be envisioned as moving in the fluid flow. It will always move tangent to the streamline when the flow is steady (does not change with time).

• *Turbulence* in a flowing fluid means that there are velocity fluctuations where the fluid changes its

Table 4.1 Water properties at various temperatures.

Temperature, T (°C)	Density, ρ (kg·m^{-3})	Kinematic viscosity, $\nu \times 10^6$ (m$^2 \cdot$ s^{-1})
10	999.7	1.304
15	999.1	1.137
20	998.2	1.002
25	997.1	0.891
30	995.7	0.798
35	994.1	0.728

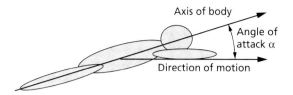

Fig. 4.1 A body moving at an angle of attack of 20°.

magnitude and/or direction. Although turbulence involves random fluctuations, it has been found by experiment that certain average properties of the fluctuations are adequate to describe turbulent flow. These two standard properties are called turbulence intensity and turbulence length or scale.

• *Turbulence intensity* may be viewed as a measure of the fluid velocity fluctuation over time relative to the steady state velocity. Mathematically it is defined as the ratio of the root-mean-square of the velocity fluctuations to the mean flow velocity. In a swimming pool during a race, swimmers will encounter turbulent water that has been churned up by themselves or other swimmers, as well as still water with little or zero turbulence.

• *Turbulence length or scale* may be viewed as the size of pockets or balls of turbulence in the water. It is likely that turbulence scale will be comparable in size to pressure wakes and vortices shed from other swimmers.

• *Angle of attack* (α) is the angle at which an object is inclined from the direction of flow. Figure 4.1 shows a body moving at an angle of attack of approximately 20°.

Dimensionless parameters of fluid mechanics

There are several dimensionless parameters that play very important roles in fluid mechanics. Four of these parameters can be applied to swimming, and they are defined next. Each parameter contains something called a characteristic length (L). This is a dimension that best describes the size of an object involved in the fluid flow of interest. Examples of a characteristic length for an airplane wing, sphere, and a swimmer's hand would be, respectively, the wing chord length, the sphere diameter, and the width of the hand (thumb to little finger).

• *Reynolds number (Re)* was developed in 1863 by Osborn Reynolds. It provides a criterion to determine the state of flow for problems where the relationship between inertia and viscous forces is important—a common occurrence in swimming. Reynolds number is defined as

$$Re = \frac{\rho v L}{\mu} = \frac{vL}{\nu} \qquad (4.1)$$

where ρ is the fluid density, v is the velocity of the fluid relative to an object in the flow field, L is the characteristic length, μ is the fluid absolute viscosity, and ν is the fluid kinematic viscosity. Two examples of Reynolds number calculations are shown below:

1 *Example*: Calculate the Reynolds number for the downbeat kick of a butterfly swimmer's foot moving at 5.5 m·s^{-1}, when the foot is 0.12-m wide and the water temperature is 25°C.

Solution: $Re = vL/\nu = 5.5$ m·s^{-1}(0.12 m)/0.891 $\times 10^{-6}$ m^2·s^{-1} $= 7.407 \times 10^5$

2 *Example*: Calculate the Reynolds number for a swimmer's hand moving at 2.4 m · s^{-1}. The hand width is 0.1 m and the water temperature is 25°C.

Solution: $Re = vL/\nu = 2.4$ m ·s^{-1} (0.1 m)/0.891 $\times 10^{-6}$ m^2·s^{-1} $= 2.694 \times 10^5$

• *Froude number (Fr)* is a dimensionless parameter that is significant for fluid flow around objects that are in proximity of, or penetrating through, a free surface. For swimming applications, the free surface is the air–water interface. The Froude number is important for wave drag, and is defined as

$$Fr = \frac{v}{\sqrt{gL}} \qquad (4.2)$$

where v is the velocity of the fluid relative an object in the flow field, g is the acceleration due to gravity (9.8146 m·s^{-2}), and L is a characteristic length descriptive of an object in a flow field, just as for Reynolds number.

1 *Example*: Calculate the Froude number for a swimmer in the streamlined position, moving at 1 m·s^{-1} with a length L, fingertips to toes, of 2.1 m.

Solution: $v = 1$ m·s^{-1}, $L = 2.1$ m, $g = 9.8146$ m·s^{-2}

$$Fr = \frac{v}{\sqrt{gL}} = \frac{1}{\sqrt{9.8146(2.1)}} = 0.22$$

• *Acceleration number* (δ) is a dimensionless parameter that can be correlated to drag resistance for conditions of acceleration or deceleration that does not involve frequency (no oscillation). The acceleration number is defined as

$$\delta = aL/v^2 \qquad (4.3)$$

where a is the constant acceleration (m·s^{-2}), L is the characteristic length (m), and v is the average velocity during the acceleration (m·s^{-1})

• *Strouhal number* (S) is a dimensionless parameter that is important when there exists some type of frequency associated with the fluid flow. The Strouhal number is defined as:

$$S = nL/v \qquad (4.4)$$

where n is the frequency of the cyclic condition (cycles·s^{-1}), L is the characteristic length (m), and v is the velocity (m·s^{-1}). For example, the Stouhal number would be important in the evaluation of a swimmer of length L moving through the water at velocity v and butterfly kicking at a frequency of n cycles·s^{-1}.

General categories of fluid motion

It is useful to classify fluid flow into categories based upon its physical characteristics. The characteristics are numerous, and they can be combined together in a variety of ways to form many categories of flow. Each unique category of flow is governed by mathematical equations that can differ greatly from one another based upon the characteristics of the flows involved. For instance, the flow of a fluid that is steady, incompressible, and inviscid (also called an ideal fluid) is represented by mathematically simple equations in comparison to those for unsteady compressible viscous flow. The mathematics will not be presented here, but the reader should conceptually understand the differences between the various types of fluid flow that are discussed next. Why is this important? This information will be helpful in understanding Chapter 5, where the drag and propulsive forces discussed depend upon the type of flow being evaluated.

• *Internal vs. external vs. open channel flow*—Internal flow is flow completely bounded by solid boundaries.

Examples are water flowing through pipes or air flowing through ducts. External flow is the unbounded flow around solids totally immersed in a fluid, such as airflow around an airplane. Open channel flow occurs when there is a so-called free surface (air–water interface) present. An example of this would be the flow of a river. The flow of water around a swimmer has characteristics from both external flow and open channel flow. While many of the fluid mechanics phenomena we will apply to swimmers come from external flow assumptions, some of them, such as wave drag, result from the presence of a free surface.

• *Steady vs. unsteady flow*—When the *time-averaged* properties at each point in a flow field do not change with time, the flow is called steady. For a body moving through water, this requires that a body's size, shape, orientation, and velocity relative to the water remain constant. The flow around a swimmer is almost always unsteady. The changes in speed and/or the direction of motion of the arms and legs are obvious, and these changes significantly affect how much propulsive force swimmers can develop. Also obvious is the change in body velocity during the breaststroke ($\pm45\%$ from the mean body velocity). But even the body velocity of an elite freestyle swimmer can vary as much as $\pm15\%$ from the mean velocity. The unsteady flow about swimmers hands and arms will be discussed at length in Chapter 5. It is important to note that a fluid can be both steady and turbulent. It is the *average* flow properties remaining constant with time that make the flow steady, and it is the microfluctuations about these average values that make the flow turbulent.

• *Compressible vs. incompressible flow*—When the density of a fluid changes, the flow is compressible. Flow is incompressible when variations in density are negligible, as is true for most flows involving swimming. One exception occurs when air bubbles are injected into the water by a swimmer's arms and legs. This phenomenon is called entrainment, and the addition of the bubbles changes the average density of the water in the entrainment area. Once the arms or legs have moved far enough to leave the bubbles behind, the flow becomes incompressible again.

The movement of the liquid–bubble mixture caused by entrainment is called two-phase flow. Two-phase flow is a very complicated subject, but one simple way to model such a mixture is to consider it a homogeneous fluid with a mass density approximately equal to that of water with a compressibility arising from the air bubble content. There have been more accurate studies that show how density varies with bubble size, air–water mass ratios, and pressure, but their application to swimming is not yet practical, mainly because we do not have quantifiable data about bubble entrainment. Also, the effective "shape" of the hand (that the water "sees") may be totally changed by bubbles temporarily adhering to the hand surface, thus changing the propulsive ability of the hand.

• *Viscous vs. inviscid flow*—Inviscid fluid flow has no viscosity. Put a swimmer in such a fluid, and there is no drag! Actually such a fluid does not really exist, but the concept can be very useful for some flow situations. For example, for fluids, such as water, that have a relatively small viscosity, the effects of internal friction in the fluid are significant only in a thin region along any boundary. For swimmers, this means that viscosity is only important for the fluid flowing very near the swimmer's skin. This area of flow is called the boundary layer. Although small in size, the boundary layer plays a large role in drag calculations (this is discussed in more detail later in this chapter). Outside the boundary layer, the flow may be considered as inviscid.

• *Uniform vs. nonuniform flow*—Uniform flow occurs when the velocity is equal at every point in the flow (equal in both magnitude and direction) at any given instant in time. The velocity can, however, change with time. Flow where the velocity varies from place to place for any given instant of time is called nonuniform. The flow of water moving around a swimmer is nonuniform.

• *Rotational (vortex) flow vs. irrotational flow*—When fluid particles in a fluid rotate about any axis the flow is called rotational or vortex flow. Otherwise, the flow is called irrotational. Flow around swimmers is, at many places, rotational. The most obvious examples are the vortices created by a swimmer's hands and feet.

• *Ideal flow*—Fluid flow that is both incompressible and inviscid is called an ideal fluid. Ideal fluids can be represented by mathematically simple equations.

• *Laminar vs. turbulent flow*—Viscous flow may be split into two subcategories: laminar flow and turbulent flow. In laminar flow, the motion is smooth and can best be understood by envisioning water flowing

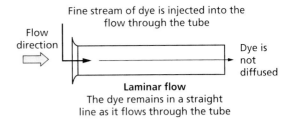

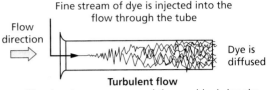

Fig. 4.2 Laminar vs. turbulent flow characteristics.

along in layers or laminae that are moving at different velocities. There is no mixing between adjacent layers; dye injected into a laminar flow would follow a single line. Turbulent flow is characterized by a mixing up of all the layers of the fluid, and dye injected into a turbulent flow would quickly break up and be dispersed among the various layers of the fluid. A comparison of the two flows is shown in Fig. 4.2. Swimmers encounter both types of flow, and whether the flow is laminar or turbulent greatly affects a swimmer's drag.

• *Boundary layer flow vs. free stream flow*—When fluid flows around an object, the object has a localized effect on the flow velocity. The fluid velocity is zero at the solid–fluid interface, and increases to what is called the free stream velocity within a thin layer of fluid immediately adjacent to the interface. This thin layer is called the boundary layer, and the flow inside it is viscous. The depth of the boundary layer varies with the pressure, velocity, and viscosity of the fluid and the shape and roughness of the object. Flow inside a boundary layer can be either laminar or turbulent. Laminar flow is generally characterized by smaller Reynolds numbers than is turbulent flow. A laminar boundary layer will get thicker as the fluid moves along the surface, and may eventually become turbulent or separated (see later). Laminar and turbulent boundary layers have different flow profiles (Fig. 4.3) that account for significant differences in drag.

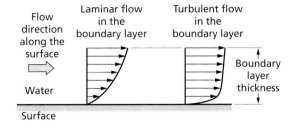

Fig. 4.3 Flow profiles of a laminar and turbulent boundary layer (looking from the side).

Outside the boundary layer, the free stream flow may be considered to be inviscid and can be split into two categories: undisturbed free stream flow, which is the flow area of the free stream that would not change whether the object was there or not, and disturbed free stream flow, which is the flow area of the free stream affected by the object, but still considered to be inviscid. Figure 4.4 shows the regimes of flow that can occur along the surface of a submerged object. As will be discussed in Chapter 5, the status of the boundary layer is critical in determining the speed of a swimmer.

For submerged objects, there is a critical Reynolds number at which the boundary layer begins a transition from laminar flow to turbulent flow. The value of this number depends on the object's surface roughness, the amount of initial turbulence in the stream, and how quickly pressure and velocity change along the length of the boundary layer. At swimming race velocities, the Reynolds numbers for various moving body parts are of the orders 10^5 and 10^6.

• *Separated vs. attached flow*—Attached flow occurs when the boundary layer follows the contours of the submerged object. If the boundary layer stops following these contours, the flow is said to be separated. The total drag on a swimmer or any object moving through water is greatly increased when boundary layer separation takes place. Engineers go to great lengths to design objects so that flow passing by them remains attached to the surface. They try to avoid separation by not making any "sudden" changes to the surface shape of the object in the flow. It is analogous to driving your car around a curve in the road. If the road curves too sharply for the speed you are traveling, your car will slide off the road. The same idea applies to water as it moves around a body. If the body curves too sharply for the velocity of the water, the water just cannot "make the curve," and will separate from the surface, creating a low-pressure area behind the object. An example of

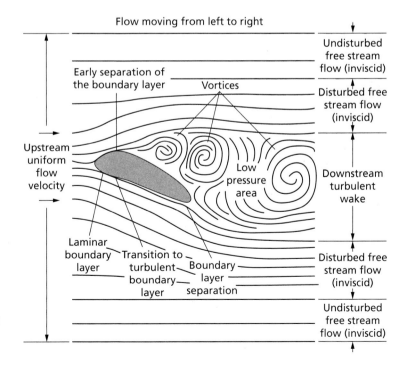

Fig. 4.4 Types of flow around a bluff (blunt) object (roughly the cross section of a palm).

this may be seen in Fig. 4.4. Because of the shape and velocity of a swimmer moving through water, there are areas where the boundary layer separates from a swimmer's body. How this separation increases a swimmer's drag will be discussed in Chapter 5.

Categories of flow that apply to swimming

The motion of a swimmer is far more complicated than even that of a fighter aircraft undergoing the most extreme maneuver possible. Indeed, in a single-stroke cycle swimmers encounter all the categories of flow listed earlier, except internal flow. This wide range of flow categories and the complex variation of flow with time and location prohibit exact closed-form analyses of the fluid flow field around a swimmer. However, in some cases, simplifying assumptions may be made to reduce the complexity of the flow problem, and allow the application of simplified fluid mechanics equations to be applied to specific parts of a stroke. When this is done, it is important to remember the assumptions (and associated limitations) that were made to allow the development of the simplified equations. These assumptions should properly be viewed as information as significant as the principles or equations themselves. Why is this obvious fact even mentioned? All too often in the published literature, theories or results valid for a specific type of flow have been broadly misapplied to all flow types. One example, discussed in Chapter 5, is the persistent misuse of Bernoulli's equation to explain the lift generated by a swimmer's hands.

Principle of relative motion for steady flow

On December 17, 1903, Wilbur and Orville Wright made history as they flew mankind's first sustained powered flight in a heavier-than-air machine. The Wright brothers were much more than a couple of bicycle mechanics—as they have occasionally been described. Their correspondence with knowledgeable engineers throughout the world and their lectures to engineering societies about aerodynamics showed them to be well ahead of other aviation enthusiasts of their time. Although they used data obtained from various gliding experiments by Otto Lilienthal and Octave Chanute, it was their own research in their own wind tunnel that contributed most to their success. They had reasoned that the aerodynamic forces on an airplane are the same whether the airplane moves through still air or the airplane is fixed and air is moved past it. In other words, it is only the relative motion of the air and the airplane that is important.

This principle is very convenient because it allows us to change our frame of reference, one moment discussing water flowing past a swimmer and the next moment discussing a swimmer moving through the water, knowing that the forces generated between the water and swimmer are the same in both circumstances. There is, however, one very important restriction to this principle: *It only applies to steady flow, and not to unsteady flow.*

For unsteady flow, the force on a stationary body in an accelerating fluid is greater than the force on a body accelerating through a fluid by a factor called the horizontal buoyancy force. The horizontal buoyancy force, so named because it is brought about by a horizontal pressure gradient, is equal to $\rho \forall a$, where ρ is the fluid density, $\forall$ is a characteristic volume of the body (similar to a characteristic length), and a is the acceleration of the body. As was noted previously, the velocities of a swimmer's hands and center of mass during the four strokes show various degrees of unsteadiness. So while the application of the principle of relative motion to a freestyler's center of gravity would result in only a small error, a similar application to the body motion of a breaststroker or the hand and arm motions for any of the four strokes would result in more significant errors. A method to account for unsteady flow in drag calculations is presented in Chapter 5.

Recommended reading

Fox, R.W. & McDonald, A.T. (1992) *Introduction to Fluid Mechanics*. New York: Wiley.
Schlichting, H. & Gersten, K. (2000) *Boundary-Layer Theory*, 8th edn. New York: Springer-Verlag.

Chapter 5
Resistance and propulsion

Barry S. Bixler

Have you ever dreamed of flying through the sky like a bird? As children, most of us had that dream at some point in our life. And even once in a while as adults, in those rare moments of uninterrupted quiet, some of us still wonder what it would be like to soar effortlessly above the earthbound masses. Astronauts achieve weightlessness of course, but they can only propel themselves by pushing off from their spacecraft wall, and then they cannot change direction or speed. The fact is—we humans do fly—not in air, but in water. We call it swimming. We propel ourselves through water without aid of machines, changing speed and direction at will, or even just "hovering" like hummingbirds at the water's surface. Swimming is the closest thing to flying (without other apparatus) that we humans will ever do, and in this chapter, we will discuss how we accomplish it.

Newton's laws of motion

The starting points for almost any subject in mechanics are Isaac Newton's laws of motion. They were formulated by Newton after carrying out a large number of experiments, and were published in the *Principia* (1686):
• First Law: A body of constant mass remains at rest, or moves with constant velocity in a straight line, unless acted upon by a force.
• Second Law: A particle acted upon by a force (F) moves (velocity v) so that the time rate of change of its linear momentum equals the force. Mathematically,

for a mass (m), which can change with time, this may be written as three equations:

$$F_i = \frac{\mathrm{d}}{\mathrm{dt}} m v_i \qquad (5.1)$$

where i represents the three principle coordinate axes.
• Third Law: To every action there is an equal and opposite reaction.

Newton's second law for swimmers

Newton's second law refers to a particle. But what happens when we have a system of particles or an extended body (not discreet particles), such as a swimmer, acted upon by forces? Assuming the swimmer is made up of a system of masses (arms, legs, head, etc.), then the center of mass (or center of gravity) of this system moves as if the total external forces applied to the system were acting on the entire mass of the system concentrated at its center of mass. Thus, the three equations of Newton's second law are still applicable. However, extended bodies also require a description of their angular motion. Three additional equations are necessary:

$$M_i = I_{i1}\frac{\mathrm{d}\omega_1}{\mathrm{dt}} + I_{i2}\frac{\mathrm{d}\omega_2}{\mathrm{dt}} + I_{i3}\frac{\mathrm{d}\omega_3}{\mathrm{dt}} \qquad (5.2)$$

where M_i are the applied torques about each of the principal coordinate axes, ω_1, ω_2, and ω_3 are the angular velocities about the three axes, and I_{ij} are the moments or products of inertia at time t.

If we know the mass and all the forces acting upon a swimmer, we can, by applying these six equations, solve for the motion of a swimmer's center of mass at any point in time. But, as we shall see in this chapter, the forces acting upon a swimmer depend upon velocity, position, and time. Their complexity makes an exact mathematical representation of them very difficult, and hence, an accurate solution to the equations of motion becomes difficult as well. It is these forces, both resistive and propulsive, that are the main topic of this chapter.

Although six degrees of freedom (three translational and three rotational) are required to thoroughly describe all possible motions of the center of mass of a swimmer, the main direction of interest is the longitudinal (forward–back) direction. Significant local *cyclic* translations and rotations by the arms, legs, head, and torso occur in all directions, but the major movement of the swimmer's center of mass is along the body's *longitudinal* axis (parallel to the lane lines). If we temporarily limit our discussion to this direction only, then the following simple equation that relates a swimmer's mass and acceleration to force may be stated:

$$\text{Propulsive forces} - \text{Resistive forces}$$
$$= \text{Mass} \times \text{Acceleration} \quad (5.3)$$

where *propulsive forces* are the longitudinal components of force generated by swimmers to propel themselves forward and *resistive forces* are the longitudinal components of force that resist forward motion.

Although this equation oversimplifies the problem in several ways, this single equation clearly shows that for swimmers to go faster, they must increase propulsive force and/or decrease resistive force. This is no great surprise, but how that is accomplished takes a little more thought. And there is one important aspect of equation 5.3 that must be remembered—seldom do swimmers generate forces in the exact direction they want to go (down the lane to the wall). Thus, force components in the direction of interest must be calculated from the overall propulsive force (Fig. 5.1). The same applies to the resistive forces.

It may be added that although we distinguish between propulsive and resistive forces, in reality, we propel ourselves through the water by creating resistive forces. We move our hands through the water,

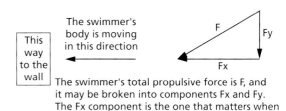

The swimmer's total propulsive force is F, and it may be broken into components Fx and Fy. The Fx component is the one that matters when calculating propulsive force towards the wall

Fig. 5.1 Components of a force.

pushing or pulling against it. The water resists this motion, and resistive forces are created. Newton's third law now comes into play, and an equal and opposite propelling force is created, moving the swimmer ahead through the water.

Drag and lift forces

When a swimmer moves through water, the water exerts a resistive pressure (always perpendicular to the body surface) and resistive shear stress (parallel to body surface) on each individual "local" part (head, arms, legs, etc.) of the swimmer's body. Pressure and shear forces acting upon each local part may be calculated by dividing the pressure and shear stresses by the areas upon which they act. Then, these forces can be resolved into components along three orthogonal (perpendicular to each other) axes. Commonly, one axis is aligned with the direction in which the local body part is moving. The force component in this direction is called *drag*, and the drag force always points in the direction opposite to which the body part is moving. The other two force components can either be combined to create a single force called three-dimensional (3D) lift (which is still perpendicular to the drag force), or remain separate as two-dimensional (2D) lift and axial force (or other description suitable to the application). This force component resolution along the three orthogonal axes is shown in Fig. 5.2. *Lift force is simply a force perpendicular to the direction of motion.* Note that this definition says *nothing* about how the lift force was created.

Since the various parts of a swimmer's body are not moving in the same direction, the "local" drag and lift forces for each part are not resolved into the same

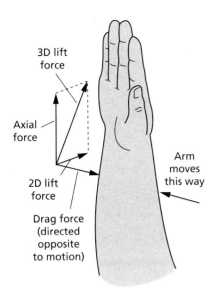

3D lift
force

Axial
force

Arm
moves
this way

2D lift
force

Drag force
(directed
opposite
to motion)

Fig. 5.2 Drag and lift force components.

coordinate system. To determine the total drag and lift forces on a swimmer's body, all local drag and lift forces should be resolved into the "global" coordinate system, which is aligned with the swimmer's motion toward the wall. A simplified 2D example of this resolution is shown in Fig. 5.3. The true resolution must, of course, be done in three dimensions.

Aerodynamic body types

Bodies moving through a fluid may be aerodynamically split into two groups: *slender bodies* and *bluff bodies*. Examples of slender bodies are flat plates or thin airfoils at zero angle of attack. Examples of bluff bodies are thick airfoils, spheres, cubes, or anything else that presents a rather broad surface to the flow around it. A slender airfoil rotated to an angle of attack of only $10°$ becomes a bluff body. A swimmer's body falls into the bluff body group. While friction drag is the major drag component on a slender body, most of the drag on a bluff body is form drag (sometimes called pressure drag). Figure 5.4 shows the percentage of total drag due to form drag for an airfoil ($Re = 4 \times 10^5$ and $\alpha = 0$) plotted vs. the ratio of the airfoil thickness (T) to the airfoil chord length (L). It is easily seen that

as the ratio of the airfoil thickness to its chord length gets larger, form drag becomes dominant, even for a very smooth airfoil. For the extremely bluff shape of a swimmer, where significant flow separation occurs, form drag is the dominant drag.

The drag and lift equations for steady flow

An exact closed form mathematical analysis of the flow around a submerged or half-submerged bluff swimmer's body is effectively prohibited by significant boundary layer separation from the body. Experimental testing has traditionally been used to estimate various drag and lift forces on a swimmer, although recently, as computers have gotten faster, a technique called computational fluid dynamics (CFD) has emerged as an alternative and supplement to experimental testing. This technique is discussed later in this chapter.

For a *totally submerged* bluff object in *steady* flow conditions and away from the water surface, the results of either an experimental test or a CFD analysis are usually plots of the drag coefficient C_D and lift coefficient C_L vs. Reynolds number. An example of such a plot, made for the drag of a cylinder, is shown in Fig. 5.5. Similarly shaped curves could be developed for any bluff object, and for swimmers and any other bluff object, they would look very similar. Note that Fig. 5.5 is a log–log plot, and that the relationship between the drag coefficient and the Reynolds number is very nonlinear. The drag and lift coefficients are defined as

$$C_D = \frac{F_D}{\frac{1}{2}\rho V^2 A} \qquad (5.4)$$

$$C_L = \frac{F_L}{\frac{1}{2}\rho V^2 A} \qquad (5.5)$$

where F_D and F_L are the drag and lift forces, respectively, ρ is the water density, V is the steady freestream velocity of the water relative to cylinder, and A is the area created by projecting the cylinder onto a plane perpendicular to the flow.

Equations 5.4 and 5.5 are based upon viscous and steady flow, and they are often introduced without qualification in the swimming literature as "the"

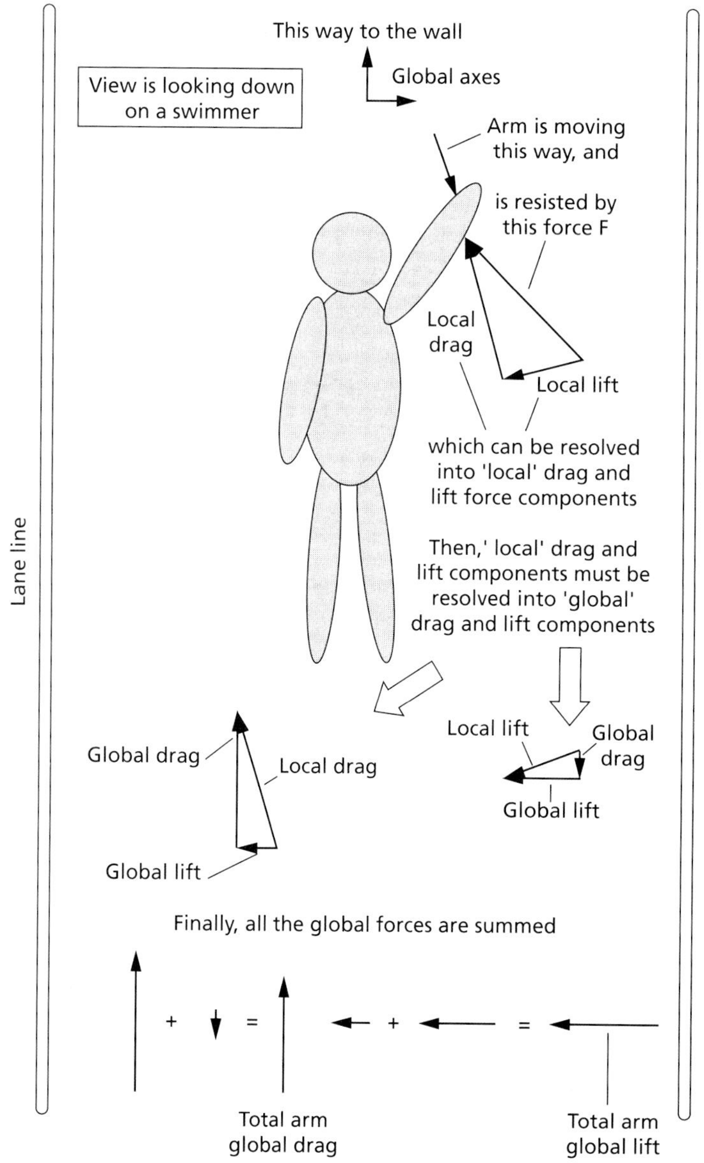

Fig. 5.3 Resolution of arm force into local drag and lift forces, and then into arm global drag and lift forces.

equations for drag and lift calculations on a swimmer. Unfortunately, their use to predict *total* drag and lift on a swimmer or on a part of a swimmer is only approximate for several reasons:
• Flow about a swimmer is unsteady, and a swimmer's acceleration and deceleration significantly affect drag and somewhat affect lift.
• Free surface effects complicate the flow by allowing wave drag and ventilation.

• Flow around a swimmer may become compressible because of local density changes caused by air bubble entrainment.

In addition, the swimming literature is full of references where, stemming from equation 5.4, a swimmer's drag is incorrectly said to be proportional to the swimmer's velocity squared. In fact, since the drag coefficient (C_D) itself depends upon Reynolds number (and hence velocity), this statement cannot be strictly

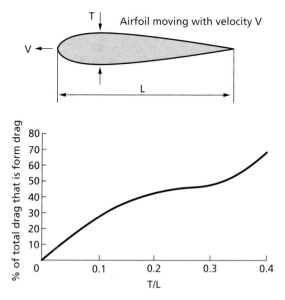

Fig. 5.4 Percentage of total drag due to form drag for smooth airfoils of various aspect ratios.

true for all velocities. However, as may be seen in Fig. 5.5, there can be limited ranges of Reynolds numbers where the drag coefficient is constant.

The quasi-steady approach to force evaluation

Realizing that flow around a swimmer is never steady, many swimming scientists have used what is called

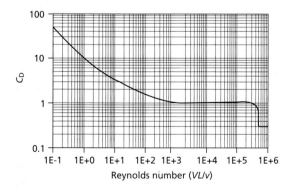

Fig. 5.5 Drag coefficient for a cylinder.

the "quasi-steady" approach to estimate hand and arm forces created by swimmers during the propulsive phase of their strokes. Drag and lift coefficients at various angles of attack for a typical hand or a hand/arm combined have been determined through experimental testing in flumes (Schleihauf 1979), tow tanks (Berger *et al.* 1995), and wind tunnels (Wood 1977), or by CFD (Bixler 1999; Bixler & Riewald 2002). Then, using video to estimate the position and velocity of the hand/arm during a typical stroke, the propulsive drag and lift force of an accelerating hand/arm has been calculated using *steady-state* coefficients for velocities at "snapshot" time points during the stroke. This technique is a good first step toward handling unsteady motion, as it takes into account the changes in velocity during a stroke. However, it ignores the inertial aspects of the unsteady motion, which can be significant.

Fluid added mass and the drag equation for unsteady flow

As a swimmer's hand moves through a stroke cycle, accelerating and decelerating, the hand experiences a drag and lift force as the water resists its motion, and imparts an equal but opposite force to the water, thus providing propulsion. Look again at Newton's second law of motion (eq. 5.3).

What is the mass *m* in equation 5.3? The answer is water and the hand mass itself. The next obvious question is, How much water? Some water is pushed by the hand and some flows around the hand. The additional mass of water pushed by the hand is called the *fluid added mass* or virtual mass, and scientists and engineers have been analyzing and experimenting for over 200 years to determine the correct added mass for various objects moving in either air or water. Obviously, added mass is more significant in water than in air because of the differences in density.

Added mass can be represented by a nondimensional *added mass factor k*, which is determined experimentally and is defined as the added mass divided by the mass of fluid displaced by the object. Research on added mass began in the late 1700s, with significant progress made by the early 1800s. Much of the early research on unsteady flow was done using symmetric objects at zero angle of attack, and the lift forces in most cases were zero. Hence, for the moment, we will focus on drag forces, although similar arguments can be made for lift forces.

It is possible to write a drag equation for unsteady flow that includes added mass, assuming a moving body is well beneath the surface (no wave-making). If a body is accelerated through water that was initially at rest, its drag at time t may be written as

$$F_D = \frac{1}{2}\rho C_D V^2 A + k\rho \forall a \qquad (5.6)$$

where ρ is the fluid density, C_D is the drag coefficient for steady-state flow, V is the instantaneous velocity at time t, A is the characteristic area of the body on which C_D is based, k is the added mass coefficient, also called the fluid inertial coefficient, $\forall$ is the characteristic volume of the body on which k is based (usually the displaced volume of water), and a is the instantaneous acceleration at time t.

The first term of equation 5.6 is recognizable as the drag due to steady-state motion. The second term represents the unsteady effects. Both C_D and k are determined experimentally. The value of k is variable and depends upon the state of motion. It is obvious that a significant testing program would be required to develop accurate and reliable added mass coefficients. Further complications would develop if k were determined by oscillating acceleration tests rather than unidirectional acceleration tests. In that case, k would also be dependent upon the amplitude and oscillation period of the test apparatus.

It is important to emphasize that equation 5.6 is valid only when there is no wave drag or compressibility. This means that it could be applied to the motion of the hand once it is well under the surface and all trapped bubbles have fallen away.

It is interesting that equation 5.6 provides a mathematical explanation as to why some coaches intuitively talk to their swimmers about "grabbing" as much water with their hands as possible. The more water that is "grabbed," the larger the added mass.

Equation 5.6 is valid for an accelerating or decelerating body in an initially stationary fluid. For fluid accelerating around a stationary body, k would be replaced by $(1 + k)$, accounting for the additional buoyancy force, $\rho \forall a$, mentioned in Chapter 4.

The acceleration number

A less complicated, alternative approach that addresses unsteady flow was developed by Iversen and Balent (1951) for unidirectional accelerating or decelerating objects (no cyclic oscillation). They determined that a dimensionless parameter called the *acceleration number* (δ) could be correlated to unsteady drag resistance. This parameter, introduced in Chapter 4, is equal to aL/V^2, where a is the constant acceleration, L is a characteristic length, and V is the average velocity through the unsteady motion.

Comparison: quasi-steady forces vs. actual unsteady forces

Riewald and Bixler (2001a, 2001b) used CFD techniques to calculate the time-dependent forces in an accelerating and decelerating hand/arm and compare them with forces calculated using the quasi-steady assumption. It was shown that even for a mild acceleration of $2 \text{ m} \cdot \text{s}^{-2}$ (with attack angle of $60°$), unsteady drag and axial forces are significantly different from quasi-steady forces, while the lift forces from both methods are more similar. This trend was also seen for other accelerations and angles.

Riewald and Bixler (2001a) also found simple relationships between the acceleration number and the ratio of the average unsteady force divided by the average quasi-steady force (during a stroke segment of constant acceleration or deceleration). These relationships allow the calculation of unsteady forces using steady force coefficients and the acceleration number. The acceleration numbers used in the analyses ranged from 0.10 to 0.45. The most disparity between unsteady and quasi-steady forces occurred for drag, where for the arms, unsteady drag could be more than twice the quasi-steady drag, and for the hands, unsteady drag could be more than 1.5 times the quasi-steady drag. One interesting discovery was that although swimmers may still be pushing backwards at the end of their stroke, if their hand and arm are decelerating too sharply, the inertia effects of the deceleration will dominate to the extent that the swimmer is producing a negative propulsive force.

The types of drag

We are interested in both drag and lift forces, but during the following discussions, we will mainly be referring to drag. This is only a matter of convenience, as many of the same principles that apply to drag also apply to lift. Also, it should again be emphasized that although we sometimes distinguish between propulsive drag forces and resistive drag forces, in reality, we propel ourselves through the water using resistive forces. We move our hands, arms, and feet through the water, pushing or pulling against it. The water resists this motion, and drag and lift forces are created. Newton's third law is applicable, and an equal and opposite propelling force is created, moving the swimmer through the water. Throughout this discussion of drag, we will switch between propulsive and resistive drag examples without comment.

Drag can be categorized in two ways. The first way is to categorize drag according to what the swimmer is doing. This gives us either *passive drag,* which is the drag swimmers encounter when their body is in a fixed position (such as streamlining off a turn), or *active drag,* which is the drag they encounter when "actively" stroking and kicking. Although active drag is the most meaningful of these two, it is impossible to evaluate analytically at the present. All approaches to date have been experimental in nature. One way (di Prampero *et al.* 1974) has been to add extra known drag incrementally to a swimmer, require them to swim at the same speed, and then measure $\dot{V}o_2$ uptake for each extra drag added. By developing an equation that relates $\dot{V}o_2$ above resting to extra drag, the active drag may be determined by extrapolating the equation to the baseline of resting $\dot{V}o_2$. Swimmers studied by Kolmogorov and Duplisheheva (1992) also towed bodies of known drag, but instead of requiring the swimmer to swim at a constant velocity, they had the swimmers swim at the maximum velocity possible. Then, knowing the difference in velocity with and without the towed weight, they assumed that the power used in both cases would be the same. That allowed them to back-calculate the active drag. Probably the best approach to date has been used by Toussaint *et al.* (1988), where using the MAD (Measuring Active Drag) system, swimmers push off from pads mounted below the surface of the water. The pads measure the force, and once the pad forces are integrated over time, they yield the average force required to overcome the active drag at the swimmer's velocity.

The other way to categorize drag is according to what is causing it (pressure, friction, waves, etc.). This way presents the most opportunities to quantify the drag, and thus will be the focus in this book.

Both pressure (normal to the surface) and shear stresses (tangential to the surface) applied by the water to a swimmer's skin and swimsuit may contribute to drag and lift. If we divide the pressure and shear stresses by the areas upon which they act, we will get normal and shear forces. Each of these forces can be resolved into local drag and lift forces, as shown in Fig. 5.6. Thereafter, the local forces can be further resolved into "global" drag and lift forces, as was shown in Fig. 5.3.

The drag due to pressure is, naturally, called pressure drag, and the drag due to a shear load is called skin friction drag. There are several types of pressure drag forces, and even among fluid mechanists there is some disagreement about how they should be categorized. Table 5.1 shows the types of drag encountered by a swimmer using the terminology most commonly employed by fluid mechanists. The first five are mutually exclusive, and the last four are alternative definitions or combinations of the others. Figure 5.7 shows how all of them are related. Sometimes all of the pressure drag is called form drag.

The dominant drag encountered by swimmers is pressure drag, although the others are also important. Form drag, skin friction drag, interference drag, and induced drag are usually associated with a Reynolds number, while wave drag and spray drag are usually associated with a Froude number. Each type of drag is discussed in detail later in this chapter.

Factors that affect a swimmer's drag

Each of the factors in Table 5.2 affects one or all of the types of drag that swimmers encounter. How this happens is discussed next. In some cases, the effect of a single factor on a single type of drag can be determined, while in other cases, it is only possible to quantify how a factor affects *total* drag.

In the following paragraphs, it is important not to confuse turbulent (but still attached) boundary

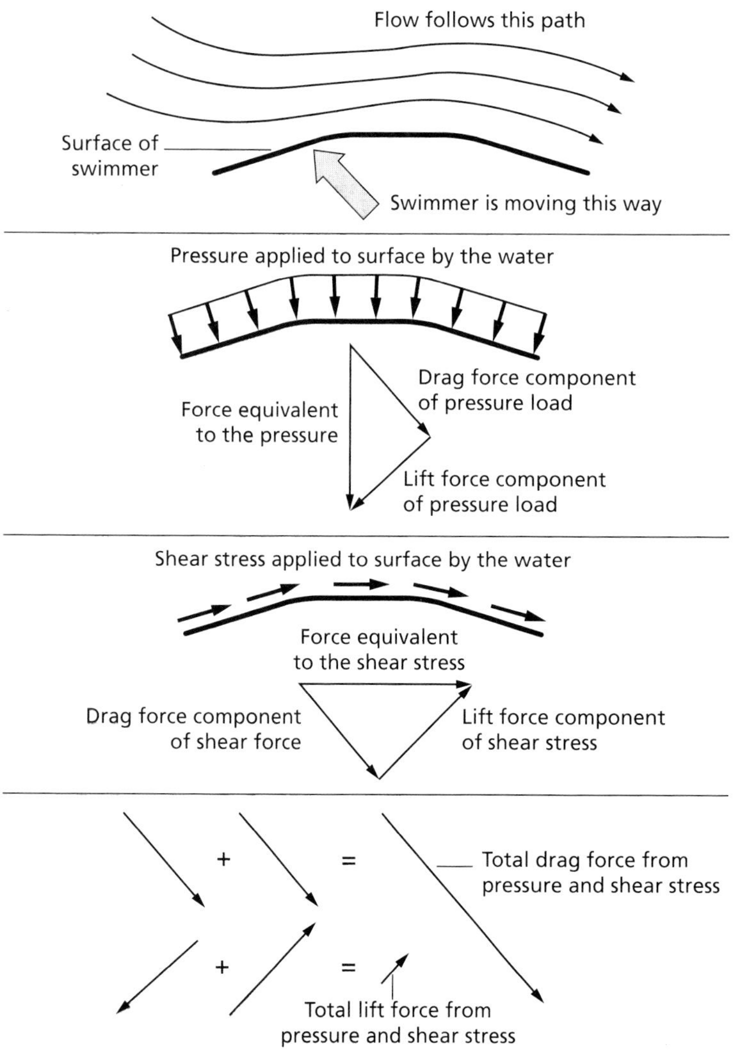

Flow follows this path

Surface of
swimmer

Swimmer is moving this way

Pressure applied to surface by the water

Force equivalent
to the pressure

Drag force component
of pressure load

Lift force component
of pressure load

Shear stress applied to surface by the water

Force equivalent
to the shear stress

Drag force component
of shear force

Lift force component
of shear stress

+ = Total drag force from
pressure and shear stress

+ = Total lift force from
pressure and shear stress

Fig. 5.6 Resolution of pressure and
shear forces into drag and lift forces.

layer flow with separated turbulent flow. And also, remember that although the word drag is used in the following discussion, in many cases, lift could be directly substituted, since lift is merely a force component perpendicular to the drag force.

Form drag

Effect of the boundary layer on form drag

The concept of a boundary layer and its separation from an object was introduced in Chapter 4. Form drag

is a viscous pressure drag caused by boundary layer separation, and for swimmers it is the most important of all the drag forces. Early boundary layer separation, as demonstrated at the top of the surface of the object in Fig. 4.4, results in large form drag and the development of a large turbulent wake area behind the object. Form drag is so named because the shape or form of an object plays a major role in determining when the boundary layer separates and what the form drag will be. To illustrate simply how form drag develops, we will look at the boundary layer flow around a cylinder. The same principles demonstrated with the cylinder apply equally to the bluff body of a swimmer.

Table 5.1 Types of drag.

Form drag	Caused by the shape and orientation of the swimmer
Skin friction drag	Caused by friction between water and the swimmer
Wave drag	Caused by the formation of waves
Spray drag	Caused by the formation of spray
Interference drag	Caused by two body parts being close to each other
Induced drag	Caused by the generation of lift
Parasitic drag	Equal to total drag—induced drag
Pressure drag	Equal to total drag—skin fraction drag
Eddy resistance	Another term for form drag (ship-building industry)

The normalized pressure distribution on the surface of a cylinder immersed in a uniform steady *inviscid* flow is plotted as a solid line in Fig. 5.8. The sum of this pressure over the surface of the cylinder resolved into the direction of motion is zero, resulting in zero drag. In fact, we know that the flow within the boundary layer is viscous, not inviscid, and the actual pressure distribution will be different, resulting in a net drag force on the cylinder.

For *viscous* flow around the cylinder, the boundary layer will begin to develop at point 1 in Fig. 5.8. As the flow moves from point 1 to point 2, the pressure on the surface decreases and the fluid accelerates. The acceleration of the fluid in the boundary layer tends to oppose the action of the viscous shear forces, resulting in the development of what fluid mechanists call a *favorable pressure gradient*. Over the rear half of the cylinder, starting at point 2, the pressure begins

to increase, slowing down the fluid in the boundary layer. This increasing pressure has the same effect on the fluid as viscous shear, developing what mechanists call an *adverse pressure gradient*. The fluid near the surface of the rear half of the cylinder now slows down, and if the adverse pressure gradient is large enough, it may cause a flow reversal. This flow reversal marks the point where the boundary layer begins to separate, as is demonstrated in Fig. 5.9. The flow reversal gives rise to vortex (whirlpool) flows in the separated region, which spin away from the cylinder, creating a wake like that seen in Fig. 4.4.

The pressure distribution on the cylinder downstream from the point of separation is radically changed by boundary layer separation. Figure 5.8 also shows the pressure on the cylinder surface *downstream* from the separation points for both laminar and turbulent boundary layers. The pressure downstream from the separation points is negative, approximately uniform, and equal to the pressure at the separation points, making the sum of the pressure on the rear half of the cylinder less than the sum of the pressure on the front half of the cylinder. The net force resultant on the cylinder is called form drag.

The single largest influence on drag is the condition of the boundary layer. In a study by Hay and Thayer (1989), the pattern of water flow around swimmers was observed by attaching small tufts of highly visible material at discreet points over the swimmers' bodies and observing the movement of these tufts. Separated flow was revealed by highly varied tuft orientation, while attached flow was apparent where the tufts were nicely aligned and lying on the body surface. In two

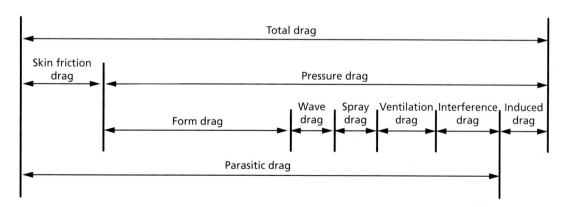

Fig. 5.7 Relationships between the various types of drag (length of line is not an absolute indicator of drag magnitude, although in general, pressure drag on a swimmer is larger than skin friction drag).

Table 5.2 Factors that affect a swimmer's drag.

Boundary layer status
Size, shape, and orientation of the swimmer's body
Velocity of the swimmer (or parts of the swimmer)
Acceleration of the swimmer (or parts of the swimmer)
Surface roughness of the swimmer and swimsuit
Water density
Freestream turbulence of the water
Temperature of the water
Submergence depth of the swimmer (or parts of the swimmer)

---

other studies by Bixler (1999) and Bixler and Riewald (2002), CFD techniques were used to reveal where the boundary layer separated from a swimmer's hand and arm, and where vortices formed on the downstream side of a swimmer's hand and arm (Fig. 5.10).

The fact that some of the flow around a swimmer is separated has significant consequences for almost all types of drag. The pressure plots in Fig. 5.8 show that a turbulent but still attached boundary layer causes less form drag than does a laminar boundary layer. The profiles of these two types of boundary layers were shown in Fig. 4.3, where it was seen that near the surface of a swimmer, a turbulent boundary layer has a greater velocity than a laminar one. This increased kinetic energy, due to turbulent mixing, enables the turbulent boundary layer to better resist an adverse pressure gradient near the surface, thus delaying boundary layer separation and reducing form drag. This explains the sudden drop in the drag coefficient seen in Fig. 5.5 at a Reynolds number of about 5×10^5. This drop is caused by the boundary layer changing from laminar to turbulent, delaying boundary layer separation, and reducing the drag force and drag coefficient. And so we come to the well-known story of how golf ball dimples increase the distance the ball will travel. The dimples trip the boundary layer, making it change from laminar to turbulent, thus delaying boundary layer separation, lowering form drag, and allowing the golf ball to travel farther. Incidentally, the dimples *increase* skin friction drag, but form drag is so dominant that the net effect is to reduce overall drag.

Effect of body shape, body size, and orientation on form drag

As the size of an object is increased, assuming the shape and orientation remain the same, the form drag is increased proportionately, with some adjustments made for the change in characteristic length in the Reynolds number. More important are the shape of an object and its orientation, for variances in these parameters can greatly affect the boundary layer.

It should now be clear that delaying the boundary layer separation can minimize form drag on any submerged object. In other words, move the point of boundary layer separation as close as possible to the rear end of the object by reducing the adverse pressure gradient acting on the surface of the object. Both in aerodynamics and swimming this process is called *streamlining*. Two extreme cases presented in Fig. 5.11 demonstrate the effect of streamlining, where a flat plate is either aligned with the flow or perpendicular to the flow. The total drag is small when the plate is aligned with the flow, with most of it resulting from skin friction. An adverse pressure gradient does not develop, there is no separation, and the form drag is negligible. When the plate is perpendicular to the flow, skin friction drag is negligible because the fluid immediately separates from the surface, and the total drag, almost all of it form drag, is very large, much larger than the skin friction drag.

A striking example that demonstrates the importance of streamlining is shown in Fig. 5.12. The two objects (an airfoil and a cylinder) have the same form drag. Although the airfoil is many times larger than the cylinder, the streamlined shape of the airfoil keeps the boundary layer from separating, thus keeping the form drag equal to that of the very small cylinder. A final and perhaps more familiar example involves the icing of aircraft wings. During adverse weather, a small layer of ice may collect along the leading edge of airplane wings, slightly changing the aerodynamic shape of the wing and causing early boundary layer separation. This greatly increases form drag and also reduces lift. It is hard to imagine that such a little amount of ice is so important, but wing icing has been responsible for more than a few airplane crashes. Although the consequences of not streamlining in swimming are not as severe, swimmers should strive to streamline their bodies at all times (starts, turns, strokes, and even finishes). Any *unnecessary* side-to-side or up and down wiggling motions should be eliminated. These motions essentially enlarge the body size that the water "sees," promote boundary separation, and increase form drag.

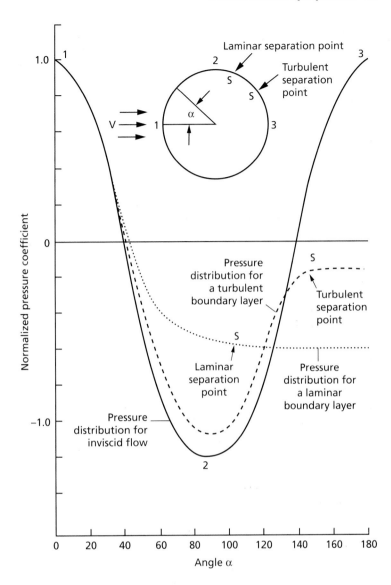

Fig. 5.8 Pressure field around a cylinder. Inviscid flow compared with laminar and turbulent boundary layer flow.

Effect of velocity on form drag

Form drag will always increase as a swimmer's velocity increases, assuming other variables remain constant, and there are no transitions in the boundary layer. There is no single mathematical formula to describe how form drag changes with velocity in all situations. For obvious reasons, swimmers should never *decrease* their velocity simply to *decrease* form drag, but rather think of *decreasing* their drag to *increase* their velocity.

Effect of acceleration on form drag

When a swimmer's arm accelerates, the propulsive drag is increased beyond steady-state drag. Likewise, when a swimmer's arm decelerates, the propulsive drag is reduced below steady-state drag. These results apply to any kind of bluff object, including a swimmer's head. They are for total drag, but a swimmer's hand and arm are so dominated by form drag, that the conclusions also hold true for just form drag. It is easy to see then that *ideally*, to maximize the drag

Water flow direction

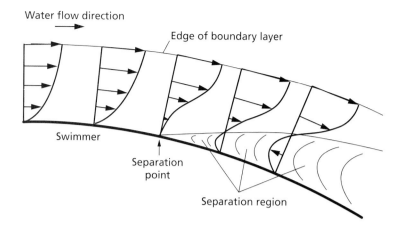

Fig. 5.9 An adverse pressure gradient causes flow reversal and boundary layer separation.

force against the stroking hands and arms (thus increasing the equal and opposite propulsive force), the hands and arms should continually accelerate during the underwater part of the stroke cycle.

Effect of surface roughness on form drag

The surface roughness of a swimmer's skin and swimsuit influence form drag in a very complex fashion. A rough surface may cause earlier boundary layer separation, thus increasing form drag. But at other times and/or locations, it may reduce form drag by causing the boundary layer to transition from laminar to turbulent flow, and delaying boundary layer separation. Surface roughness effects on form drag in swimming have never been quantified, but they are probably insignificant compared to some of the other factors discussed in this section. The same cannot be said about some other sports, where the effect is greater and is easier to quantify. The golf ball dimples are a classical example.

Effect of water density on form drag

If the water next to a swimmer's hand is entrained with air, then the density and pressure of the water in the area of entrainment may be changed, thus affecting the form drag. Entrainment may initiate an early boundary layer separation, causing an increase in the

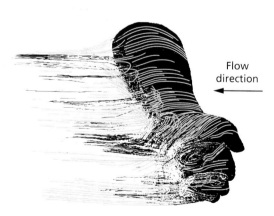

Fig. 5.10 Flow path lines around a swimmer's hand and arm show significant boundary layer separation.

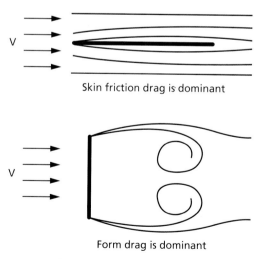

Skin friction drag is dominant

Form drag is dominant

Fig. 5.11 How body orientation affects drag.

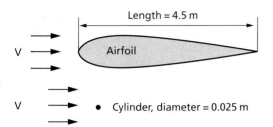

Fig. 5.12 Two objects that have approximately equal form drag.

form drag. Or, if the entrainment is substantial, it may "round out" the hand, changing it to be more streamlined, and making it less able to generate propulsive force. Until the entrainment can be quantified, nothing more can be concluded.

Effect of freestream water turbulence on form drag

Freestream water turbulence, defined in Chapter 4, can be represented by two parameters, turbulence intensity and turbulence scale (or turbulence length).

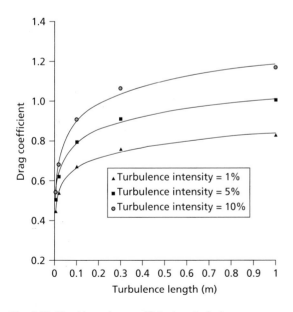

Fig. 5.13 Hand/arm drag coefficient vs. turbulence parameters. Angle of attack = 45°, velocity = $2m \cdot s^{-1}$, and drag coefficient is based upon the maximum projected area.

Form drag increases with increased water turbulence. A swimmer's drag moving through initially turbulent water is higher than when moving through undisturbed water. Bixler (1999) studied the effects of water turbulence on propulsive drag using a CFD model of a hand and arm, and found that form drag increases if either of these parameters is increased (Fig. 5.13). As points of reference, the flume at USA Swimming in Colorado Springs has a turbulence intensity of 4% and a turbulence scale of about 0.1 m, while the larger flume at the University of Otago in New Zealand has a turbulence intensity of 1% and a turbulence scale of 0.093 m.

Effect of water temperature on form drag

The *total* drag of a swimmer is affected by water temperature in two ways. First, the drag force in equation 5.4 is directly proportional to the density, and since increases in temperature decrease density, increases in temperature will also reduce drag. These changes are very small however, compared to the effect that temperature has on viscosity, because viscosity changes as much as 15% within the range of water temperatures encountered by swimmers (see Table 4.1). As water temperature increases, viscosity decreases, and total drag decreases. What proportion of this decrease should be attributed to form drag is not known, because viscosity plays a role in several types of drag.

Effect of submergence depth on form drag

The submergence depth of a swimmer, or parts of a swimmer, affect drag because the nearness of the free surface (air–water interface) influences the flow field around the swimmer. It is difficult to quantify the effect depth has on form drag, but it may be confidently stated that an object moving along the surface encounters less form drag (but more wave drag) than an object moving well beneath the surface. There are three reasons why this occurs:

1 There is less underwater body surface upon which a pressure exists.

2 The elevation of the water surface changes in response to pressure changes underwater.

3 The pressure field may be modified continually or cyclically through a process called ventilation. *Ventilation* occurs when the pressure in the low-pressure region behind a submerged object falls below atmospheric pressure, and air is sucked into that region to make a cavity. This process has the effect of reducing the pressure differential between the front and back of the object, thus reducing the form drag.

Skin friction drag

Skin friction drag is the drag on a swimmer resulting from viscous shearing stresses being applied tangent to the wetted surface of a swimmer's body. Conceptually it is comparable to the friction between two solid surfaces sliding along each other.

Effect of the boundary layer on skin friction drag

The boundary layer has a critical effect on skin friction drag, opposite to its effect on form drag. Skin friction is zero where the boundary layer has separated. A bluff (non-streamlined) body will experience less skin friction drag than a streamlined one because of earlier boundary layer separation. In spite of this, the swimmer should always streamline to minimize form drag, because any decrease in skin friction caused by non-streamlining will always be overshadowed by the accompanying increase in form drag. If the boundary layer has *not* separated, skin friction drag for a laminar boundary layer is much less than for a turbulent boundary layer.

The tufts study by Hay and Thayer (1989) revealed that the attached boundary layers of significance on a swimmer's body occur on portions of relatively flat body surfaces such as the torso and thighs. Solutions for skin friction drag on flat surfaces were among the first boundary layer problems solved at the beginning of the twentieth century. The boundary layer solution developed by Blasius (1908) for steady incompressible *laminar* flow parallel to one side of a smooth flat surface and valid for Reynolds numbers up to approximately 5×10^5 is

$$F_{\mathrm{D}} = 0.664 b\rho \sqrt{\nu L V^3} \qquad (5.7)$$

where F_{D} is the total skin friction drag on the surface, b is the surface width, L is the surface length, ρ is the mass density, ν is the fluid kinematic viscosity, and V is the velocity outside the boundary layer.

Equation 5.7 may also be written using the form of equation 5.4, containing a *friction* drag coefficient C_{f}.

$$F_{\mathrm{D}} = C_{\mathrm{f}} \left(\frac{1}{2} \rho V^2 A \right) \qquad (5.8)$$

where $C_{\mathrm{f}} = 1.328/\sqrt{Re}$, A is the wetted area of the surface, and Reynolds number (Re) is based upon the length of the surface.

It is also possible to determine the skin friction drag when a boundary layer is turbulent. Equation 5.9 is valid for steady incompressible turbulent flow parallel to one side of a flat surface, and for Reynolds numbers between approximately 5×10^5 and 10^7 on smooth surfaces. The variables are defined the same as they are in equation 5.7.

$$F_{\mathrm{D}} = 0.036 b\rho \nu^{-1/5} L^{4/5} V^{9/5} \qquad (5.9)$$

Equation 5.8 may also be written with a *friction* drag coefficient as

$$F_{\mathrm{D}} = C_{\mathrm{f}} \left(\frac{1}{2} \rho V^2 A \right) \qquad (5.10)$$

where $C_{\mathrm{f}} = 0.074/(Re)^{-1/5}$, A is the wetted area of the surface, and Reynolds number (Re) is based upon the length of the surface.

Friction drag coefficients for both laminar and turbulent boundary layers are plotted in Fig. 5.14 as a function of Reynolds number. In the development of

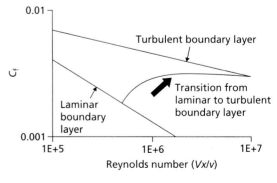

Fig. 5.14 Skin friction drag coefficient vs. Reynolds number (Re) (based upon surface distance x).

equation 5.8 it was assumed that the boundary layer is turbulent from the leading edge of the body onwards. In fact, in a pristine flow environment, the boundary layer will initially be laminar and then transition to turbulent further downstream. For smooth surfaces the point of transition will occur around a Reynolds number of 5×10^5. The curved line between the laminar and turbulent boundary layer is typical for a transition event. However, this curve is for an ideal situation. Swimmers encounter turbulent water and make sudden accelerations and decelerations both forward and laterally, making it likely that the point of transition will occur at a lower Reynolds number. In fact, the transition will occur almost immediately, and there will be almost no laminar flow.

Equations 5.6 through 5.9 were for flat smooth surfaces at zero angle of attack with zero pressure gradients. This is an ideal situation, but provides a technical base upon which to build our knowledge of skin friction drag. Turbulent boundary layers in the presence of a positive or negative pressure gradient along a surface are beyond the scope of this book, but Rota (1962) provides a good summary of the work performed in this area.

Effect of body shape, size, and orientation on skin friction drag

The shape and orientation of a body affect the skin friction drag by influencing the boundary layer. Any non-streamlined body shape or orientation that causes early boundary layer separation will minimize skin friction drag. The effect of body size on skin friction drag along flat smooth surfaces may be quantified with the use of equations 5.7 through 5.10. Laminar and turbulent frictional drag are proportional to $L^{1/2}$ and $L^{4/5}$, respectively. In other words, doubling the surface length of a swimmer does not double the skin friction drag. This occurs because the downstream part of the surface has a thicker boundary layer, resulting in lower friction drag than on the upstream portion of the surface.

Effect of velocity on skin friction drag

As with other types of drag, skin friction drag is greatly affected by the relative velocity of the swimmer to the water. Equation 5.7 for *laminar* flow along a flat surface shows that the skin friction drag is proportional to (Velocity)$^{3/2}$, while equation 5.9 shows that the skin friction drag for a *turbulent* boundary layer is proportional to (Velocity)$^{9/5}$.

Effect of acceleration on skin friction drag

As with form drag, it is difficult to isolate the effects of acceleration on a single type of drag. The only thing we can say for certain is that, assuming no transition in the boundary layer occurs, the skin friction drag will increase as acceleration occurs.

Effect of surface roughness on skin friction drag

The surface roughness of a swimmer's skin and swimsuit can affect the skin friction drag. A rough surface results in greater skin friction drag than a smooth surface, provided that other factors remain constant. For this reason, some swimmers have started wearing "fast" suits. A separate section devoted just to the Fastskin swimsuits introduced by Speedo during the last Olympics is presented later in this chapter. These suits have generated a tremendous amount of interest as well as controversy, and the manner in which they have been designed to reduce friction drag will be presented.

Sharkskin or not, the time-honored tradition of shaving off body hair prior to a big meet still continues everywhere. Although it has been theorized that shaving increases performance only by enhancing kinesthetic sensitivity or "psyching up" the swimmer, a study by Sharp and Costill (1989) appears to show otherwise. They found that swimmers who shaved typically had an increase in performance. Although it may be true that skin friction drag is smaller than form drag, friction drag is significant nevertheless.

Once a boundary layer transitions from laminar flow to turbulent flow (but is not yet separated), the influence of surface roughness on skin friction drag is important only after the Reynolds number reaches a certain value. If an object is moving at a given speed V, then a *permissible surface particle size* **k** or *depth of roughness* on the object's surface may be calculated (do not confuse this **k** with the added mass coefficient k). The permissible surface particle size represents the maximum roughness a surface may have before beginning to influence turbulent friction drag. For Re within the swimming range (less than 10^6), the following very simple equation relates **k** to Re and ℓ, the length of the boundary layer (Schlichting 1987).

$$\mathbf{k} = \frac{100\ell}{Re} \qquad (5.11)$$

To get a feeling for what **k** means, several values of **k** (in mm) for familiar surfaces are as follows: glass, 0.0001; galvanized metal, 0.152; raw wood, 0.51; concrete, 1.27.

Now let us consider the following example, which is very ideal, but effectively demonstrates the influence of surface roughness on turbulent boundary layer flow. Research has shown that most swimmers have an attached turbulent boundary layer along their stomachs. If swimmers move at a steady speed of $2 \text{ m} \cdot \text{s}^{-1}$, a typical boundary layer length on the stomach is observed to be 0.25 m long. If the water temperature is $20°C$, what is the maximum permissible roughness a swimsuit (or a stomach) can have before beginning to influence turbulent friction drag?

Solution: For a water temperature of $20°C$, $v = 1.02 \times 10^{-6} \text{ m}^2 \cdot \text{s}^{-1}$

$$Re = VL/v = 2\text{m} \cdot \text{s}^{-1}(0.25 \text{ m})/1.02 \times 10^{-6} \text{ m}^2 \cdot \text{s}^{-1}$$
$$= 5.1 \times 10^5$$

From equation 5.11, $\mathbf{k} = \frac{100\ell}{Re} = 100(0.25)/5.1 \times 10^5 = 0.00005 \text{ m} = 0.05 \text{ mm}$.

This is the theoretical roughness below which a swimsuit (or skin) may be considered as "smooth." In other words, if a swimsuit or a swimmer's skin has a roughness greater than 0.05 mm, then this roughness will contribute to turbulent friction drag. Exactly how this surface roughness is defined and determined is obviously very important, but the various procedures to accomplish that are beyond the scope of the present discussion.

Since the 0.05-mm roughness is meaningful only for *turbulent* skin friction, the question then becomes: In those areas where the boundary layer is attached to the swimmer's body, is the flow laminar or turbulent? The value of the critical Reynolds number where the boundary layer transitions from laminar to turbulent depends on surface roughness, the amount of freestream turbulence, and how quickly pressure and velocity are changing along the length of the boundary layer. Typical transition Reynolds numbers range between 2×10^5 and 4×10^5 for blunt objects and approximately 5×10^5 for flow along flat surfaces. These numbers would be reduced to 1×10^5 or less for situations with significant freestream turbulence.

Since swimmers do indeed encounter a lot of freestream turbulence from other swimmers and from themselves, a likely critical Reynolds number for boundary layer transition would be around 1×10^5 or even less. Therefore, in areas where the flow is still attached to a swimmer's body, the boundary layer becomes immediately turbulent, and consequently, friction drag will be influenced by any surface roughness greater than the critical roughness.

Effect of water density on skin friction drag

As shown by equations 5.7 and 5.9, skin friction drag is directly proportional to water density for both a laminar and a turbulent boundary layer.

Effect of water temperature on skin friction drag

Water temperature affects skin friction through its effect on viscosity (which varies with temperature). For laminar and turbulent boundary layer flow, the skin friction drag is proportional to $v^{1/2}$ and to $v^{-1/5}$, respectively. The relationship of v to water temperature was given in Table 4.1.

Effect of freestream water turbulence on skin friction drag

A change in freestream turbulence can affect when the boundary layer transitions from laminar to turbulent, which in turn affects the skin friction drag as previously described.

Effect of submergence depth on skin friction drag

If submerged parts of a swimmer are close enough to the free surface to be affected by ventilation, then where ventilation occurs, the skin friction will drop to zero.

Wave drag

Swimmers encounter two types of waves: *external waves*, created by wind or other swimmers, and *internal waves*, created by themselves.

External waves

Although external waves may be dampened by lane lines, they still can create a choppy and turbulent water surface. In general, as the water gets rougher, swimmers' times get slower. There are four ways by which rough water may slow down a swimmer:

• The fluid flow field (pressure and velocity) around a swimmer is abruptly changed when a swimmer meets a wave. This represents an increase in random turbulence of the freestream flow, which, as we saw earlier, results in increased drag.

• The waves deform the water surface so that hands, head, legs or even the torso enter into the water at different angles and at different instants in the stroke cycle than when the water surface is flat and not moving. The entries into the water by various parts of the body are not as "clean," and extra splash or spray is created. Spray represents another form of drag, which will be covered in the next section.

• Waves encountering a swimmer are reflected off the swimmer in a similar way they are reflected off walls. The reflection of these waves requires energy, thus representing drag.

• Additional slowing may also occur if the swimmer's stroking rhythm or "feel" for the water is "thrown off" by encountering a rough water surface.

There have been many studies, tests, and analyses of wave drag by the shipbuilding industry, and some of them are applicable to swimmers. Ikegami and Imaizumi (1979) conducted experimental and analytical investigations on the speed loss of model ships in irregular waves and in regularly spaced waves of wavelength λ (distance between crests). They found that the additional drag from external waves is usually significant only when the ratio of λ/L, where L is the ship length, is between 0.5 and 2.0. They also found that maximum speed loss occurred when λ/L was equal to 1.0.

Waves generated by swimmers generally have a wavelength of 1.3 m or less, with taller swimmers generating waves with the largest wavelengths. If the length of a swimmer is 1.8 m, then $\lambda/L = 0.72$, well within the range of where external waves can increase drag. Although pool swimmers will fortunately not encounter waves with wavelengths as long as their bodies, open water swimmers may definitely be affected by such large waves.

Internal waves

The other types of waves encountered by swimmers are internal (self-generated) waves. The creation of these waves takes energy, and that energy is supplied by the swimmer. Thus wave-making is also a type of drag. The pattern of internal waves is predictable, and is shown in Fig. 5.15. The earliest analytical account of these types of waves comes from Lord Kelvin (1887), who observed them emanating from ships and modeled them as a single pressure point traveling over the surface of the water. Although very simple, the Kelvin wave explains many of the features of waves generated by moving objects, including swimmers.

The V-shaped waves shown in Fig. 5.15, called *diverging waves*, emanate from the swimmer's body at an angle from the direction of motion, much like the waves generated by a ship. Fast swimmers usually generate either two or three of these waves, depending on the swimmer, the stroke, and the speed. The most prominent of these is the first bow wave, so called because it corresponds to the wave generated at the bow (forward tip) of a ship. The bow wave emanates from a point at the front of a swimmer's head.

The other kind of self-generated waves, also shown in Fig. 5.15, are called *transverse waves*. They move in the same direction as the swimmer, and stretch

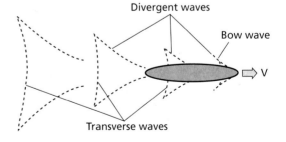

Fig. 5.15 Overhead view of diverging and transverse waves behind an object moving along the surface of the water.

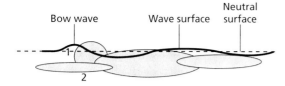

Fig. 5.16 Free water surface responds to pressure changes, creating a wave.

transversely across the path that was taken by the swimmer. These waves have a wavelength twice the wavelength of the diverging waves. Ships also have this type of wave, and they can be easily seen directly behind a moving ship. Although swimmers generate similar transverse waves, they are usually obscured by the turbulence created by stroking, kicking, the rolling motion of the torso in the freestyle and backstroke, and the up and down motion of the torso during the breaststroke and butterfly. In fact, these torso movements themselves create additional waves and spray, contributing to the total wave drag. The transverse waves behind a swimmer are best seen when the torso and arm movements are small, such as when a swimmer kicks through the water while holding onto a kickboard or keeping the hands in front of the body.

Figure 5.16 shows a swimmer's head half submerged and moving through the water. In a similar fashion to the submerged cylinder shown in Fig. 5.8, the maximum pressure on the head occurs at the front of the head (point 1). The normalized pressure on the head then drops as the water accelerates laterally around it, and becomes negative between points 1 and 2. Thus, wave drag from the bow wave appears in the form of a net longitudinal component of the pressure distribution along the head. The "free" water surface responds to these pressure changes. The high pressure at the front of the head pushes the water up, creating the bow wave. Then, where the normalized pressure drops, the water level drops and moves below the "normal" level. This "trough" behind the bow wave may permit swimmers to breathe during the freestyle without turning their heads as much as if the water surface were at the normal level. The remainder of a swimmer's body, because it is attached to the head, also affects wave drag, but it is the bow wave that is most visible.

Firby (1975) noted that some swimmers generate two sets of diverging waves while others generate three, depending on the swimmer and the stroke. The diverging waves from two-wave swimmers emanate from their head and their hips, while waves from the three-wave swimmers emanate from their head, hips, and ankles. Firby also noted that shorter freestylers tend to be two-wave swimmers, while taller ones tend to be three-wave swimmers. Additionally, he observed that the same swimmer would produce different wave patterns at different speeds.

Firby's observations can be explained using principles of physics. The wavelength λ of diverging waves emanating from an object moving through water is known to be

$$\lambda = \pi V^2 / g \qquad (5.12)$$

where V is the relative velocity of the water and the object, and g is the acceleration due to gravity ($9.8146 \, \mathrm{m \cdot s^{-2}}$).

For a freestyle swimmer of height 1.9 m and moving at a velocity of $1.7 \, \mathrm{m \cdot s^{-1}}$, the wavelength of the diverging waves would be $(3.1416)(1.7)^2/9.8146 = 0.92$ m. In other words, starting at the head and moving toward the feet, a wave will emanate from the body approximately every 0.9 m. Since the swimmer is 1.9 m tall, three sets of waves will be seen. A swimmer only 1.7 m tall would emanate only two sets of waves because the third wave would normally start at $2 \times 0.92 \, \mathrm{m} = 1.84 \, \mathrm{m}$ from the top of the head, a distance longer than the swimmer's height. This explains why shorter swimmers tend to emanate two waves while taller ones emanate three.

Naval architects have experimentally determined wave drag coefficients C_w for specific shapes that penetrate the free surface of the water. They are usually given as a function of the Froude number, which was defined in Chapter 4 as

$$Fr = \frac{V}{\sqrt{gL}} \qquad (5.13)$$

The Froude number is used because the main forces at work during the formation of waves are inertia and gravity forces. Once the Froude number of an object is known, then the steady-state wave drag may be determined from the wave drag equation.

$$F_\mathrm{w} = C_\mathrm{w} \left(\frac{1}{2} \rho S V^2 \right) \qquad (5.14)$$

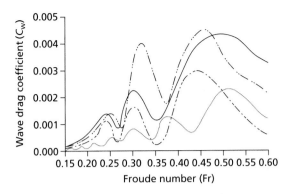

Fig. 5.17 Typical wave drag coefficients for ships.

where S is the wetted surface area of the object and C_w is the wave drag coefficient that is a function of the Froude number.

Typical relationships between C_w and Fr for various ships are shown in Fig. 5.17. Note that there are humps and valleys in the curves. These are caused by interference effects between the different waves coming off the ship. As velocity is changed, the wave profiles change, sometimes adding together to increase wave drag, and other times partially canceling each other out to decrease wave drag.

Although the magnitude of the wave drag coefficients for a swimmer could be different than those for a ship, the general form taken by the drag, with its humps and valleys, will be very similar. In the swimming literature, wave drag has often incorrectly been said to be proportional to V^3. In fact, this is what we can say about a swimmer's wave drag:

• Below a Froude number of 0.2, wave drag is relatively insignificant in comparison to total drag, and is proportional to V^2.
• Up to a Froude number of 0.4, the transverse waves are mainly responsible for the humps and valleys (Wigley 1931).
• Above a Froude number of 0.4, the contribution from the divergent waves becomes more important (Wigley 1931).
• Between Froude numbers of 0.3 and 0.4, wave drag usually increases sharply, becoming more important.
• The wave drag coefficient peaks approximately at a Froude number of 0.5, and thereafter falls away. It eventually *theoretically* drops to zero, but the reality is that above 0.5, the waves begin to break up and turn into spray (see the following section on spray drag).

Wigley showed that overall, ignoring the humps and dips in the wave drag curve, the *average* wave drag is approximately proportional to the object mass multiplied by V^6. Considering equation 5.14, wave drag then is proportional to C_w^4. Wigley (1934) also showed that the mathematical expression for steady-state wave-making resistance is of the following form:

$$F_w \propto V^6 \text{ (constant term + 4 oscillating terms)}$$
(5.15)

It is worthwhile to pause and consider the shape of the wave drag coefficient curves in Fig. 5.17. Wave drag does not monotonically increase. There are "local" valleys where, with the right combination of velocity and swimmer body length, the wave drag drops to a local minimum. Swimmers moving with the right combination of body length and velocity could have a Froude number that would put them in one of these valleys. If so, they might find that they expend *more* energy to maintain a *slower* velocity, if that velocity moves their Froude number out of a local valley.

So then, what is the Froude number of a swimmer? An age group swimmer who is 1.37 m tall and swims at velocity of 1.53 m · s^{-1} has a Froude number of

$$Fr = \frac{V}{\sqrt{gL}} = 0.42$$

A senior swimmer who is 1.8 m tall and swims at a velocity of 1.9 m · s^{-1} has a Froude number of

$$Fr = \frac{V}{\sqrt{gL}} = 0.45$$

Figure 5.17 indicates that these two swimmers would have approximately the same amount of wave drag, although the senior swimmer is moving 1.33 times faster than the age group swimmer. This is only possible because the senior swimmer is tall enough to keep the Froude number the same as the age grouper. Now let us examine how individual factors affect internal wave drag.

Effect of body shape, size, and orientation on wave drag

Body length is obviously important because of its inclusion as a part of the Froude number, and equation 5.13 shows that wave drag is proportional to the surface area of a swimmer. Thus, both swimmer length and width affect wave drag. Designers of ships that will operate at high Froude numbers make them as long and thin as possible to reduce wave-making.

Orientation of a swimmer's head, chest, and arms will also impact wave drag. Indeed, if you have ever seen breaststrokers who keep their torso inclined at an angle of attack to the water, you will have witnessed the creation of some very large waves. If the angle of attack is large enough, the swimmer will actually generate waves that emanate forward from the body, greatly increasing the swimmer's drag. This is exactly what happens with flat-faced barges as they are towed slowly through water.

Effect of velocity on wave drag

Velocity, like the length of a swimmer, is a critical part of wave drag because of its inclusion as a part of the Froude number. Although the swimming literature to date contains some research relating wave height to velocity and energy, no experimental or analytical work has been undertaken to develop curves of C_w vs. Fr for swimmers.

Effect of acceleration on wave drag

As we have already seen, swimming is usually an unsteady process. Many authors in the ship building industry have published results that show how wave drag varies with acceleration, and in some cases, wave drag was *reduced* from steady-state conditions by as much as 30% in *accelerated* flow. Efimov *et al.* (1967) compared different rates of acceleration, and found that wave drag *decreases* as acceleration *increases* for Froude numbers between 0.3 and 0.6. Thus, acceleration affects wave drag in a manner opposite to how it affects other types of drag. The same trends would be expected for swimmers.

Effect of surface roughness on wave drag

The surface roughness has a negligible effect on wave drag.

Effect of water density on wave drag

Water density affects wave drag by its role in equation 5.14. Water density can only be significantly changed through air entrainment, and as mentioned previously, that effect is difficult to quantify.

Effect of water temperature on wave drag

Only through its effect on density and viscosity can water temperature affect wave drag. Since density varies only slightly with temperature, water temperature has a negligible effect on wave drag through changes in water density. Many researchers in the field of naval architecture have attempted to examine the effects of viscosity on wave drag. Most efforts have shown that viscosity affects wave drag significantly only for low Froude numbers ($Fr < 0.2$), and even then, they are of secondary importance (Wigley 1962).

Effect of freestream water turbulence on wave drag

The freestream turbulence has a negligible effect on wave drag.

Effect of submergence depth on wave drag

An object moving underneath but still near to a free water surface will still generate wave drag. As the object gets farther away from the surface, wave drag diminishes rapidly and then disappears altogether. Research on the wave drag of slender spheroidal bodies moving at various distances under the water's free surface has shown that wave drag becomes zero once the spheroid depth is greater than five times the width (Hoerner 1965). If we were to apply this to a swimmer who is 0.40 m wide at the shoulders, then that swimmer needs to be at least 2 m under the surface of the water before *all* wave drag disappears. In fact, since the wave drag asymptotically approaches this depth, its magnitude is significantly diminished at only a depth of 1 m. A study by Lyttle and Blanksby (2000) showed that a swimmer need be only 0.6 m under water to eliminate most of the wave drag.

It is possible that the generation of wave drag may be desirable at some point during a swimmer's stroke. For example, consider the hand and arm during the backstroke. At times during the stroke the arm is moving parallel to and near to the surface. If the arm gets too close to the surface, you can see wave drag develop. If the arm gets closer still, then ventilation and/or spray drag will occur, with a lessening in water resistance to the arms motion. It is possible (but not yet known) that there is an optimum depth for moving the arm and hand where the combination of propulsive form and wave drag is actually greater than just form drag alone.

Spray drag

Spray represents another type of drag because it takes energy to splash water into the air. Although significant amounts of spray are made by swimmers, spray drag has hardly been mentioned in the swimming literature to date. There are two kinds of spray generated by swimmers: *steady-state spray* and *impulsive spray*. We will discuss these two types of spray separately.

Steady-state spray drag

This type of spray is generated steadily over a period of time, and occurs when waves made by a swimmer (or any streamlined surface-piercing object) break apart into a spray. It may be viewed as an extension of wave drag. This process starts at about a Froude number of 0.5 (Hoerner 1965) for surface-piercing objects. An object with a Froude number greater than about 3.0 creates a significant amount of spray, and the drag of this spray can be rationally calculated, as summarized by Hoerner (1965). However, the spray drag of objects with Froude numbers between 0.5 and 3.0 are difficult to predict. Since the Froude number for the body of a fast swimmer is usually around 0.5 or less, swimmers have small steady-state spray drag compared to fast-moving ships. However, if you look closely at the bow wave in front of a swimmer, you will see some spray on the peaks of the wave, especially during the sprints.

Impulsive spray drag

This type of spray is called impulsive because it is created during an instant of time as a result of a sudden dynamic event. Examples would be an arm or hand slapping the water during entry, kicking feet, or the hand stroking too closely to the water's free surface, creating a splash of water. Impulsive spray drag for swimmers is almost always cyclical. Although a swimmer's Froude number is not large enough for significant full-blown steady-state spray drag to occur, the same cannot be said of impulsive spray drag. Indeed, almost all the splash and spray seen around swimmers' hands, arms, and legs may be classified as impulsive spray, caused by the sudden movement of parts of a swimmer's body either into or out of the water. However, even less is known about this impulsive spray drag than is known about steady-state spray drag. Most of the information available comes from very simplified (and inaccurate) analyses done using inviscid irrotational flow theory, or from testing done during World War II and the 1950s when there was a flurry of government-sponsored research on water entry of bombs and missiles. Although much of the government research is now unclassified, it was done, unfortunately, for Froude numbers much larger than those of a swimmer.

Interference drag

Hydrodynamic interference occurs when the flow around an object is changed by the presence of one or more nearby objects. The interference occurs when the pressure fields of two objects interact with each other, resulting in a total net drag that is different than the sum of the separate drag values. This increment in drag is called interference drag, and its magnitude can be large. Swimmers encounter two kinds of interference drag. *External interference* occurs when one swimmer swims near another, while *internal interference* occurs when one part of a swimmer's body passes near another part of the same swimmer's body.

External interference

This usually happens when a swimmer swims in a turbulent wake created by another swimmer. It is also called *drafting*. The wake area is characterized by a pressure lower than the surrounding undisturbed water, and offers less resistance to another swimmer moving into this area. Drafting can result in a smaller pressure differential between the forward (head) and aft (toes) portions of the drafting swimmer, resulting in less form drag. A study at ICAR by Troup (1990) showed that a drafting swimmer typically expends only 94% of the energy he or she would expend if swimming alone.

The aerospace industry has done many tests to determine the interference drag of various objects. Although the drag coefficients from these tests should not be directly applied to swimmers, the trends in the tests are worth noting. The results of one study by Zdravkovich and Pridden (1977) are shown in Fig. 5.18, where the drag on a cylinder downstream from another cylinder is plotted. Both in-line drafting and offset drafting were evaluated, and the results show significant drag reductions in the downstream cylinder's drag coefficient based upon its vicinity to the leading cylinder. Naturally there were no lane lines in their experiment, and the obvious question to ask is: How well does a lane line floating on the surface of the water prevent the low-pressure turbulent wake behind a swimmer from reaching into adjacent lanes? According to the study by Troup (1990), there appears to be justification for trying to drag off swimmers in

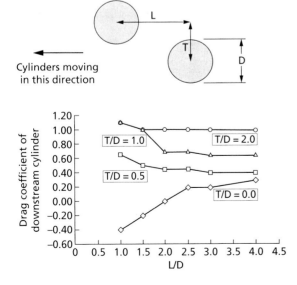

Fig. 5.18 Drag coefficient for a drafting cylinder.

an adjacent lane if they are swimming too close to the lane lines. It is important to realize that a swimmer's wake is 3D, stretching beneath the water's surface, and lane lines will not screen out the wake effects that are beneath the surface.

Another study presented in Hoerner (1965) for a pair of aerodynamically smooth struts shows that the downstream strut experiences only increased drag. So why are the two experiments giving exactly opposite results? The answer rests upon the fact that the Biermann and Herrnstein tests were made using shapes where a single strut would have very little boundary layer separation. But with struts in tandem, the leading strut created a turbulent flow for the downstream strut, causing the boundary layer of the downstream strut to separate much earlier than it normally would. This early separation increased the form drag greatly (up to a factor of 4 times), and overshadowed any decrease in drag owing to an initially lower pressure field created by drafting. On the other hand, the Zdravkovich and Pridden tests were made with bluff cylinders where the boundary layer separated early, whether there was one cylinder or two. Consequently, the boundary layer was not a factor, and the effects of the pressure differential due to drafting may be clearly seen.

So which of these two tests would apply to swimmers? The answer lies somewhere in between both sets of data—swimmers will never achieve a negative drag from drafting as in some cases of the Zdravkovich and Pridden study. But neither does drafting increase a swimmer's drag by up to four times the normal amount, as in the Biermann and Herrnstein study. These results demonstrate once again the importance of the boundary layer and the importance of understanding the assumptions made behind any equation, principle, or experiment.

Finally, one important point usually forgotten is that for the right amount of separation between two objects moving together, the drag on the leading object may also be reduced.

Internal interference

This type of interference occurs during every single stroke of any kind. Some examples of this type of interference include the legs kicking in close proximity to each other, the arms sliding along the chest at the beginning of the breaststroke recovery, the arms and hands next to the body during the butterfly and freestyle upsweep and release, the arm alongside the head during backstroke hand entry, and the hand and arm near the body just prior to release. There are many other examples that could also be mentioned.

There are two types of internal interference drag. The first kind is called *transient internal interference drag*, and for swimmers, it involves body parts moving relative to the water and also moving relative to each other. All the examples listed earlier are of this type. This type of interference drag is very difficult to determine, and certainly it has not been studied for swimmers. The second kind, called *steady-state internal interference drag*, is easier to determine, and results from one object being permanently near another object (their relative location to each other does not change).

For the moment, let us look at an example from the aerospace industry of steady-state internal interference drag. Keys and Wiesner (1975) evaluated the effects of placing an engine next to the body of a helicopter. They found that the drag on the engine was almost doubled if the engine was placed immediately adjacent to the helicopter body, but if the engine was at least half of the engine diameter away from the helicopter body, then the interference drag dropped to zero. This is obviously a huge difference, and it demonstrates how important interference drag can be.

Transient internal interference drag exists in swimming, but it has not yet been investigated or even mentioned in the literature. It could very well be, for example, that swimmers would get maximum propulsion by holding their hands and arms in certain ways when they moved close to the other body parts. But unfortunately, until research is done, we can say nothing else.

Induced drag

Induced drag is the drag that is directly associated with lift generation on a 3D object. The word "induced" comes from the similarity of the fluid flow pattern to the magnetic field pattern induced by conductors of electric current. There are many ways to calculate induced drag, and the subject can quickly get complex. We will limit our discussion in this chapter to just a few simple concepts, and refer the interested reader to the literature for more advanced treatment. It is obvious

that the only parts of a swimmer capable of generating lift are the hands, arms, legs, and feet. Therefore, induced drag pertains only to those body parts.

As a first example, let us use the smooth airfoil shape shown in Fig. 5.19 to demonstrate how induced drag is generated. Note that the airfoil is inclined from the direction of freestream flow by the angle of attack α. Since the direction of the resultant velocity at the aerodynamic center of the airfoil is tilted downward from the direction of the freestream flow by the angle α_1, the lift on the airfoil is tilted by the same angle. This effectively gives the lift vector a small component of force parallel to the freestream flow. This is the induced drag force, as shown in Fig. 5.19.

Induced drag may easily be calculated for smooth wing shapes with attached flow. But what happens when that wing approaches an angle of attack of 20°, or when it is shaped like a hand instead of a wing? That's right—the boundary layer separates. So while Fig. 5.19 provides a nice understandable picture that demonstrates what induced drag is, it is not applicable to swimming. Several techniques, most of them from the aerospace industry, have been developed to handle induced drag in complex flow situations. Schemensky (1973) provides an overall guide, where the flight domain is broken into seven regions, each of which is governed by different equations or methods to predict induced drag. Three of these regions may be applicable to swimming, as they occur in the subsonic flow domain. The three regions are distinguished by where the boundary layer separates, and whether it reattaches or not. Although the details of this study are beyond the scope of this book, the interested reader is referred to the aforementioned paper, as well as to a book by Rom (1992), which is devoted to just high angle of attack aerodynamics.

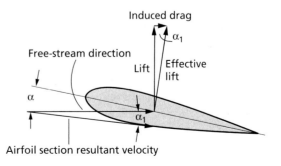

Fig. 5.19 Induced drag.

Lift

Most of the factors that cause the drag forces discussed in the last section also cause lift forces. For example, the same pressure and skin friction that create a drag component of force will also create a lift component. The same principles are at work—only the force is in a different direction. For unless an object moving through water is symmetrical and it is moving along its plane of symmetry, there will be lift generated. And even then, if the object moves far enough, a series of vortices will be shed into its wake, resulting in the generation of alternating positive and negative lift forces.

There has been confusion about lift in the swimming literature, and much of it stems from an incorrect perception of what lift is. *Lift is simply a force perpendicular to the direction of motion.* Lift occurs in many places and on many things. Lift is what tears a roof from a house during a hurricane. Lift is what causes a baseball to curve. Stick your hand out of the car the next time you drive and align it with the flow. There will be very little lift on your hand, and most of the wind force will be trying to push your hand backwards. Now turn your hand to a 45° angle with the wind direction, and feel the difference. Depending upon which way you rotated your hand, it not only wants to move backwards (drag), but it also wants to move either up or down. This is also lift. Lift is NOT limited to just the simple attached flow around an airplane wing that causes circulation and generates a lift force. That is one simple form of lift which is not applicable to swimming. There are many other forms of lift. To define lift merely as the upward force on an airplane wing would be like saying that the only type of vehicle in the world is a child's wagon, and ignore cars, boats, trains, airplanes, etc. They are all vehicles, but they provide transportation in entirely different fashions.

Bernoulli's principle

The type of lift generated by an airplane wing at small angles of attack may be mathematically described by Bernoulli's equation. For more than 30 years, the idea that Bernoulli's principle (or equation) can be used to explain the lift forces generated by swimmers has been widely accepted by the swimming community. Bernoulli's equation may accurately be applied only to fluid flow that is incompressible, inviscid, and that flows along a streamline. In fact, as has been shown by both experiment (Ferrell 1991) and analysis (Bixler 1999), the flow moving over a swimmer's hand separates from the hand on the downstream side of the hand, clearly violating the inviscid flow assumption.

The fact that Bernoulli's equation is not mathematically appropriate to describe the flow around a swimmer's hand does not mean that a swimmer does not generate lift, for lift is indeed generated. As we have seen earlier, lift is not limited to situations governed by Bernoulli's equation. The lift generated by swimmers requires more advanced equations and principles to describe it. The proper equations, well-known to fluid mechanists, are called the Navier-Stokes equations, and they govern the motion of compressible viscous fluids. The Navier-Stokes equations are complex partial differential equations, but even when they are simplified for incompressible flow, they are still too difficult to solve for most situations.

The best way to think about lift is in the most general terms possible, going back to Newton's laws of motion. When a swimmer moves a hand in a certain direction, there will be a reactive force to that motion. This reactive force is rarely directly in line with the direction of motion and is composed of both drag and lift force components. The drag component is opposite to the direction of the motion, and the lift component is in a direction perpendicular to the motion. Since a swimmer's hands move in complex patterns, both drag and lift will always contribute to a swimmer's propulsion. The big question then becomes: How should swimmers move their hands and arms to obtain the maximum propulsive force (toward the wall) from a combination of drag and lift forces. The section on propulsion will offer some insight to that question and others. But before tackling propulsion, there are a couple of interesting side issues worth addressing that occasionally you will hear being discussed at poolside.

"Fast" pools

Some pools or even some lanes in the same pool just seem "faster" than others—but are they really? The answer is a definite yes, and here are several reasons why:

• *Currents*—Some badly designed pools have currents in them that occur because of the way the water filter inlets and outlets are placed. For instance, in a certain Arizona long course pool, to remain nameless, Lane 1 has a visible current going in one direction and Lane 7 has a visible current going the opposite direction. This can make a difference in the 50-m freestyle.

• *Wind*—If a pool is located in a windy area and is not adequately sheltered, then wind can add to the external wave drag that is generated by other swimmers. Got whitecaps?

• *Lane lines* can make a difference too, for if they are not large enough, swimmers will encounter more external wave drag from other swimmers.

• *The design of both end and sidewalls* affects the reflection of waves from those walls. Plain walls without gutters will reflect more waves, as will sidewalls without lane lines strung beside them. The result is more external wave drag.

• *Water depth* is a reason often given for a pool being "fast," and this we will examine in more detail. Ideally, a swimming pool is large enough so that the progress of a swimmer is not affected by anyone or anything. This is a good idea, but we already know that external wave drag and wakes from other swimmers can affect performance, as can the end and sidewalls of the pool. Can a pool be so shallow that it affects how far a swimmer glides after a dive or a push off the wall, or even how fast a swimmer moves on the surface? Turning for answers to mainstream engineering we find the answer is yes, and in fact there are three ways a shallow pool can affect a swimmer's performance:

1 *Ground effect* is a special case of interference drag. Ground effect occurs when a moving object, by getting too close to a large fixed object such as a wall or "the ground," sees a change in its drag and/or lift forces. Pilots know about it, as lift increases just before airplanes touch down on the runway, effectively cushioning their landing. Designers of cars and high-speed trains also must consider the ground effect on lift as well. In addition to affecting lift, a "ground" surface can also affect drag, as was seen earlier with the interference drag example of the helicopter and the engine. So, if a pool is very shallow, and a swimmer gets too close to the bottom surface of the pool on the start and

on the turns, it is possible that both resistive drag and lift will be increased.

An interesting sidelight concerning ground effect involves butterfly kicking near the bottom of the pool. One possible technique that might account for the propulsion swimmers achieve when butterfly kicking is the creation and use of a series of vortices shed from their feet. This will be discussed in more detail in the section on leg and feet propulsion, but it is mentioned here because if a swimmer kicks too near the bottom of the pool, there may be some type of "ground" effect on the kicking propulsion. The magnitude of that effect is difficult to quantify without further research. Since the width of a vortex wake behind a swimmer can be as large as 1.5 m, to avoid ground effects during the butterfly kick would require a pool to be 2 m deep, giving the swimmer some margin to operate within a depth band of 1 ± 0.25 m. Some coaches are convinced that the ground effect can have a negative effect on butterfly kicking propulsion, and have trained their swimmers to perform their underwater butterfly kicks on their side, such that the vortices shed from their feet do not encounter the bottom of the pool.

2 *Blockage* occurs when an object being tested in a wind tunnel, tow tank, or a flume is too large relative to the passage that contains it. For example, consider a model ship held stationary in a shallow flume. The passage is effectively partially blocked where the ship is held. The flow cross-sectional area around the ship is reduced from what it is both behind and in front of the ship. In order to keep the same amount of water moving through the flume, the water passing under the ship must temporarily speed up more than if the ship were in deep water. Although this need is lessened if there is no restriction on the flow width (as if the ship were in a flume with sidewalls far removed), some blockage will still exist, and it will increase the drag on the ship. To avoid this, naval architects believe that the cross-sectional area of the ship or any other object should not exceed 1/200th of the cross-sectional area of the passage that contains it. If we apply this suggestion to a swimmer whose average submerged cross-sectional area is $0.08\ m^2$, the cross-sectional area of the water beneath the swimmer should be at least $16\ m^2$. If the lane width is 3 m, then the depth required to avoid blockage is 5.4 m. Since the 5.4-m number was calculated for passages with sidewalls, and the sidewalls play a critical role in blockage research, a reduction from

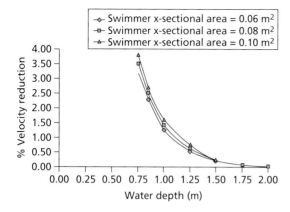

Fig. 5.20 How a swimmer's velocity is affected by water depth.

5.4 to approximately 2.0 m would seem reasonable for swimmers moving in lanes with no sidewalls.

3 *Increased wave drag* occurs in shallow water. On the basis of theory and model experiments, Schlichting (1934) determined the effect of shallow water on the wave drag of ships. His research was in shallow water with no lateral restrictions (walls). Using his data, it is possible to estimate how a shallow pool will affect a swimmer's velocity. Figure 5.20 shows how water depth would affect a swimmer who swims at 2 m · s^{-1} in water of unlimited depth. It is seen that wave drag is not affected when the water depth is 2 m or more. Thus, to eliminate either flow blockage or an effect on wave drag, the pool depth should be 2 m or more.

To plane or not to plane

Occasionally you will hear a coach or swimmer talk about *planing* on the water. Planing means skimming over the surface of the water, rather than plowing through it. It is true that some swimmers might ride slightly higher or lower in the water than others. Differences in body density could account for that. Planing, however, is a different matter entirely. To accomplish such a feat would be wonderful, but a swimmer must reach a Froude number of around 4.0 to do it. That clearly will not happen, as such a Froude number would require a swimmer to swim the 50-m freestyle in approximately 4 s.

The fluid mechanics of swimsuits

After Speedo introduced the Fastskin swimsuit during the 2000 Olympics, there was a deluge of exclamations and accusations, and political maneuvering by more than a few members of the world swimming community. Everyone had an opinion, informed or not, about the suits. The clamor was deafening to those of us who were interested. Some claimed the swimsuits were bogus—how could a fabric on your skin possibly lessen your drag? Others claimed the suits gave their wearers an unfair advantage. The surface of the Fastskin suit was designed to mimic the skin of sharks, and there was even an environmental group outraged that swimsuits were being made out of real sharkskin. Although the concerns of the environmental group have been assuaged, there is still much discussion about the suits. There has, however, been very little said about how the suits are technically designed to reduce drag. And that is the scope of the present discussion—purely technical. For the moment, leave your prejudices, politics, financial concerns, and swimming rules behind.

Sharkskin

The scales of a shark are complex. Called dermal denticles, they begin as a stem that rises out of the skin and then spreads out to lie leaf-like above the skin of the shark. They are small and closely packed together, looking something like paving stones, as seen in Fig. 5.21. The top surface has three to seven ridges aligned in the direction of flow. The average size of the scale of a fast-moving shark can range between 0.2 and 0.6 mm in length, with variances in size and shape from species to species and even from one location to another on the same shark.

Riblets

In the mid-1960s, aerodynamicists began to experiment with surfaces that contained fins or microscopic surface grooves similar to those seen in fast-swimming sharks. These grooves are called riblets. The initial research by Liu *et al* (1966) was followed with work by Walsh and Weinstein (1978). In the decades that followed, many papers were published on the subject, which showed that riblets can reduce *skin friction* drag by as much as 6–8% if the riblets are of the right size and

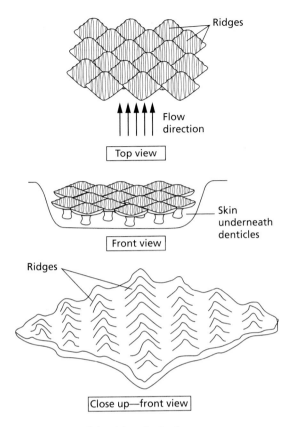

Fig. 5.21 Dermal denticles of a shark.

shape, and have the right spacing for the flow conditions. The optimum height of riblets changes with velocity and other parameters. Note that the drag reduction applies to only skin friction drag, not total drag.

Riblets have been successfully used on aircraft and missiles, and have been particularly popular in many highspeed sports such as luge sleds, racing yachts, and race cars. And now, most recently, Speedo has incorporated them into its Fastskin swimsuit. Of course, one important question is how much of a swimmer's drag is from skin friction, for it is only that portion of the drag that can be reduced by the riblets. Recent CFD analyses by Bixler (2004) of a male and female swimmer in the streamline position have shown that skin friction drag accounts for between 1/4 to 1/3 of a swimmer's total drag while underwater. Females generally also have lower skin friction drag than males. This occurs because the female shape is typically more curved than the male shape, causing earlier boundary layer separation, and hence less skin friction drag. However, even if skin friction represents only 20% of

a swimmer's total drag, and that 20% is reduced by 3%, this still gives a total drag reduction of 0.6%. In a world where victories are won by only hundredths of a second, a 0.6% reduction becomes significant. Note that this is a 0.6% reduction in drag *force*, not velocity.

How do riblets reduce skin friction drag? There are several theories, but the view most commonly held is that riblets make the turbulent flow along the surface more ordered. Water is channeled along the grooves, and cross-flow between grooves is lessened. This has the effect of hampering the development of vortices that form in the innermost part of the boundary layer right next to the surface. These vortices must move a bit farther away from the surface to form, lessening the water contact with the surface. This reduces the shear stress, and therefore the drag along the surface. Figure 5.22, which shows cross sections of a surface with riblets, demonstrates how both riblet shape and size can affect the amount by which that drag is reduced.

Another way that swimsuits have been improved is by designing the seams and even the swimsuit fabric patterns to follow the path that the water takes as

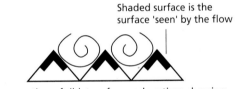

Cross-section of riblet surface and vortices, showing optimum size shape of riblet to minimize drag (flow direction is into the page)

Riblets that are not the right shape actually increase drag. Note that the area in contact with the flow is now bigger than just a flat surface

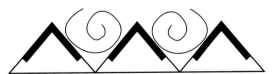

Riblets that are too big actually increase drag. Even though the vortices cannot reach the acute angles, the total area in contact with the flow is now bigger than just a flat surface

Fig. 5.22 How riblet shape and size affect drag reduction.

it flows along the swimmer's body. Speedo has done this using the results of the full body CFD analyses of Bixler (2004). Since the seams "stick up" from the regular swimsuit surface, their alignment cross-wise to the water flow could have caused premature boundary layer separation and increased form drag, as previously discussed.

Now let us come back to the swimsuit manufacturers themselves. Some have actually used science to come up with their swimsuits, but most, as is obvious from their advertising, simply have just jumped on the "full-body" bandwagon, with no real science behind their design. In fact, at least one company has even put their athletes through testing, with no intention of examining the results. Rather the purpose was to get "high-tech" pictures for promotional opportunities, and claim they did sophisticated testing. Such behavior is irresponsible, bad for the sport of swimming, and, putting it bluntly, dishonest. So, buyer beware, and hopefully this book will allow you to better determine which companies are honest, and which are simply trying to snooker you with high-tech words and pictures.

Propulsion

Although we distinguish between propulsive forces (forces used to propel us down the pool) and resistive forces (forces that resist motion in that direction), in reality, we propel ourselves by creating resistive forces. We move our hands and feet through the water, pushing or pulling against it. The water resists this motion, and resistive forces are created. According to Newton's third law of motion, an equal and opposite force is created, moving the swimmer ahead through the water. It is important to remember that swimmers do not have to move their hands and legs directly backwards to obtain an effective forward propulsive force. Indeed, the variety of stroke "styles" seen at the elite level of swimming tells us that there is more than one way to reach the wall.

The motions of a swimmer's arms and legs are usually described relative to the swimmer's body or relative to the water. The former, used by coaches, is the most practical way to instruct a swimmer how to move, while the latter is used when necessary to identify the propulsive forces involved.

In competition, swimmers can swim the backstroke, breaststroke, butterfly, and freestyle. For the freestyle, swimmers can swim any way they want to, as long as they obey a few simple rules such as touching each wall, and not touching the bottom or grabbing the lane lines. Although occasionally a swimmer may, for instance, swim the butterfly during a freestyle race, almost always swimmers use the front crawl in their freestyle races. In fact, the terms freestyle and front crawl have become so synonymous that if you asked a group of young swimmers about the crawl stroke, at least some of them would not know what you are talking about. With that in mind, the front crawl will herein be referred to as the freestyle.

Arm motions of the four competitive strokes

Recommended reading for detailed descriptions of each stroke is the classic text *Swimming Fastest* by Ernie Maglischo (2003). Although the purpose of the present book is not to teach swimming, but rather to show how the principles of science and engineering can be applied to swimming, it is still worthwhile to briefly introduce the four "sweeps" of swimming, as defined by Maglischo:

1 *Outsweep*: The initial underwater sweep in the butterfly and breaststroke
2 *Downsweep*: The initial underwater sweep used in the freestyle and backstroke
3 *Insweep*: The second sweep used in all the competitive strokes
4 *Upsweep*: The final sweep of the freestyle and butterfly

The outsweep is the first underwater motion for the butterfly and breaststroke where swimmers move their hands and arms into a position from which to begin stroking. There is little, if any, propulsion associated with this motion, where the hands are moved outside the shoulders in preparation for making "the catch." The catch is the point in a stroke where swimmers "catch" the water and start using it to propel themselves forward.

The downsweep, also mostly a nonpropulsive sweep, is the first underwater motion for the freestyle and backstroke. Like the outsweep for the butterfly and breaststroke, it gets the swimmers' hands to the point where they make their catch. However, swimmers who rotate their hand relative to their arm, as described earlier, might generate some propulsion in this sweep.

The insweep is the second sweep for all of the strokes, following the outsweep in butterfly and breaststroke, and following the downsweep in the freestyle and backstroke. It is the first propulsive sweep for the freestyle, butterfly, and breaststroke.

The upsweep is the final sweep for the freestyle and butterfly, where the hand is moving outward and upward toward the water surface.

Hand and arm propulsion

The complexity of the four swimming strokes becomes apparent after considering how many sweeps there are, and how the speed and direction of swimmers' hands and arms change during the path of a single arm stroke (Maglischo 2003). For example, the freestyle has three different sweeps, and the backstroke has even more. Complicating the issue is the changing orientation of the hand relative to the forearm, the forearm relative to the upper arm, the upper arm to the chest, and so on.

From previous discussions in this chapter, we know that the boundary layer separates from the hand and arm at the velocities (or Reynolds numbers) associated with swimming. This qualifies the hand and arm as bluff objects, where the dominant propulsive force will be form drag (and form lift). Thus, many of the principles covered in the section on drag and lift can provide us with a better understanding of how swimmers use their hands and arms for propulsion. A summary of the various aspects of the hand and arm that affect propulsion are shown in Table 5.3 and are discussed in more detail in the following paragraphs.

Table 5.3 Aspects of the hand and arm that affect propulsion.

Size of the hand and arm
Shape of the hand and arm
Orientation of the hand and arm
Location of the hand and arm
Direction of the stroke
Velocity of the stroke
Acceleration of the stroke

Effect of size and shape of the hand and arm on propulsion

Swimmers cannot control the size of their hands and arms, but they can control the shape of their hands. Since form drag and form lift are dominant, swimmers should make their hands as flat as possible. Cupping them or curving them lessens the propulsive force generated. Some swimmers hold their thumb away from their fingers (*abducted*), while others keep it next to their index finger. Research by Schleihauf (1979) has shown that when the thumb is widely separated from the plane of the fingers, the lift coefficient of the hand is larger and peaks at a lower angle of attack than when the thumb is held adjacent to them. Thus, swimmers who use a significant amount of lift force for propulsion may find that an abducted thumb will increase their propulsion.

In the same study, Schleihauf also determined that a hand with fingers slightly apart (6 mm or less) offered equal propulsive drag as when the fingers were held together. Beyond a 6-mm gap, the propulsive drag was reduced. However, for propulsive lift, any amount of gap between the fingers lessened the force. Thus it appears that the best approach for most swimmers would be to keep the fingers together.

Takagi *et al.* (2001) determined drag and lift coefficients experimentally by using an array of pressure sensors around a model of a hand. And although the coefficients were larger than those determined by other researchers (see next section), the data showed, like Schleihauf's data, that an abducted thumb can create larger lift forces at low angles of attack.

Effect of stroke direction on propulsion

The stroke direction, combined with the orientation of the hand and arm, determines what "shape" the water sees, thus affecting form drag. Together they also determine how the propulsive force is split into drag and lift components. This will be discussed further in the section on orientation.

Swimmers do not always move their hand, forearm, and arm in exactly the same direction, and the direction they stroke changes, sometimes gradually, and sometimes suddenly. There are several possible reasons why these changes occur:

1 As swimmers move their hands through the water, the water resists the motion, but because the water is not solid, it is set in motion by the hand. This water, once moving, offers less resistance to the moving hand, and it has been theorized that swimmers must either accelerate their hands to keep getting resistive force from this water, or find "still" water that will offer more resistance. The still water is found by changing the direction their hands are moving.

2 It is possible that because of changes in body position in the water, the most comfortable stroking direction may change during a stroke.

3 Changing direction may improve the swimmer's "balance," as they not only move their arms and legs, but also rotate their body. In fact, a portion of the hand and arm motion may be caused by body roll, and may not be from a conscious effort by the swimmer.

4 Swimmers lengthen the distance their arms and hands travel by not moving them straight back through the water. This allows them to get more distance per stroke.

Effect of orientation of the hand and arm on propulsion

Orientation is how the hand and arm are positioned relative to the direction of motion. Orientation, combined with stroke direction, obviously plays a large part in how much propulsion a swimmer generates. These aspects have been thoroughly investigated for steady flow conditions by Wood (1977), Schleihauf (1979), Berger *et al.* (1995) Bixler (1999), Bixler and Riewald (2002), and others.

Wood (1977) determined the drag and lift coefficients for a human hand and arm using a wind tunnel. He used four different hand and arm models of very different shapes, and the arm portion of the model extended to approximately halfway between the wrist and the elbow. He avoided boundary interference from the sting support, and although he prevented end effects with an attachment plate, forces were measured only in two dimensions (2D lift). The maximum projected area was used as a reference for force coefficient calculations.

Schleihauf (1979) evaluated a model of a hand in a flume with moving water. He accounted for the drag of the support arm, but like Wood, he calculated only 2D lift coefficients. Also, he did not adjust for the interference drag between the hand and the support. The water turbulence was unknown. The reference

area used for the force coefficients was the maximum projected area. Schleihauf's study was especially useful, since after determining the coefficients, he used video to estimate the position and orientation of a swimmer's hand during the various strokes. Then, he calculated actual forces using the hand orientation and assuming quasi-steady flow conditions. And although it has since been shown that unsteady motion of the hand creates forces well beyond those estimated by the quasi-steady approach, the quasi-steady approach was the natural first step to take, and Schleihauf's investigation was thorough, examining many different variables.

Berger *et al.* (1995) towed two different models of a hand and arm through a tow tank. By varying the depth of their models, they evaluated forces for both hand alone and hand/arm combined. For a reference area, they used the total wet surface area. They evaluated forces in three dimensions. However, their model pierced the surface of the water, creating wave drag as well as ventilation, which probably somewhat altered their force coefficients.

Bixler (1999) used the CFD model discussed previously to evaluate the force coefficients for the hand, the arm, and the hand/arm combination. This model, shown in Fig. 5.10, evaluated the effects of velocity, angle of attack, and water turbulence on drag, 2D lift, axial, and 3D lift forces and force coefficients.

The results from these four studies have been compared, and in general there is good agreement of the results. To illustrate these results, drag and lift coefficients calculated from CFD analysis for just the hand are shown in Fig. 5.23. Turbulence obviously makes a difference in drag, while it is less important for lift.

Depending upon its position, the thumb is capable of acting as a forward slat does in a slotted wing. Commercial aircraft have slats that are projected in front of the main wings during landing and takeoff. These slats, as well as the rear flaps, prevent or delay boundary layer separation up to much larger angles of attack, so that larger lift coefficients can be obtained. This does not mean, however, that a hand should ever be likened to an airfoil. In fact, the difference between an airfoil and a hand can be seen easily in what aerodynamicists call a polar diagram, which is a plot of the lift coefficient vs. the drag coefficient for different angles of attack. Figure 5.24 presents a polar diagram for both a low aspect ratio wing and a swimmer's hand,

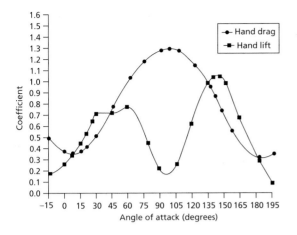

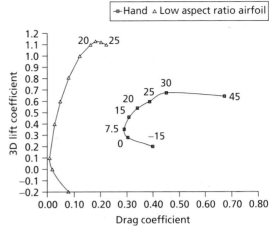

Fig. 5.23 Comparison of (a) hand drag and (b) hand lift coefficients from CFD analysis (coefficients calculated using maximum projected cross-sectional area, 5% turbulence intensity).

Fig. 5.25 A polar diagram comparison reveals that a hand is aerodynamically very different from a low aspect airfoil (angles of attack are noted in figure).

where it is easily seen that the hand and airfoil are aerodynamically very different.

Bixler also quantified how combinations of stroke direction (or stroke angle) and orientation (angle of attack) influence hand and arm propulsion. Stroke angle is defined in Fig. 5.25, where the viewpoint is above the stroking hand (cross section of the fingers is shown) as it moves through the water. Both positive and negative stroke angles are demonstrated. Also shown is the angle of attack, which is used to describe the orientation of the hand.

For each stroke angle between −90° and +90° (in 15° increments), the resultant hand propulsive force (toward the wall) was calculated for angles of attack between −15° and +195°. From these calculations, the angle of attack that provided the largest propulsive force for each stroke angle was determined. Then, the sum of the stroke angle plus the angle of attack was plotted against the stroke angle for the hand. This sum indicates the orientation of the hand relative to the long axis of the swimmer's body, with 90° representing the palm facing directly toward the feet. This

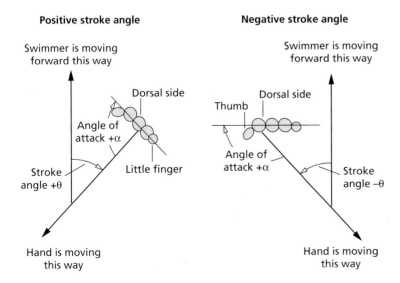

Fig. 5.24 Definition of stroke angles. The swimmer's view of the right hand for positive and negative stroke angles (looking down on the hand as it passes underneath).

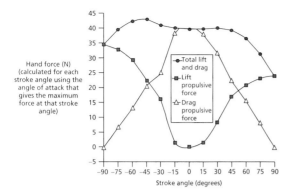

Fig. 5.26 Maximum hand propulsive force vs. stroke angle. Velocity = 2 m · s^{-1}, turbulence intensity = 1%, turbulence length = 0.1 m.

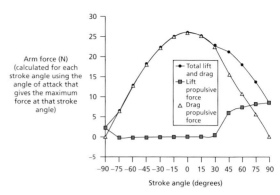

Fig. 5.27 Maximum arm propulsive force vs. stroke angle. Velocity = 2 m · s^{-1}, turbulence intensity = 1%, turbulence length = 0.1 m.

analysis revealed an important fact: for stroke angles between −45° and +45°, the maximum hand propulsion is obtained when the sum of the stroke angle and angle of attack is approximately equal to 95°. In simple terms, this means that to maximize hand propulsion, the palm should be facing directly backwards, toward the feet, for any stroke angle between −45° and +45°.

Now to the most important question: What stroke angle provides the most hand propulsion? As an example, Bixler plotted peak hand propulsive force against stroke angle for a hand velocity of 2 m · s^{-1} and a turbulence intensity and turbulence length of 1% and 0.1 m, respectively. For each stroke angle, the angle of attack that gave the largest propulsive force was used. This plot, shown in Fig. 5.26, shows that a broad range of stroke angles (between −75° and +45°) provide effective propulsion (provided the proper angle of attack is used with each stroke angle). Furthermore, the propulsive hand force varies little in this range of stroke angles, although there is a slight peak for a stroke angle of −45°.

Also shown in Fig. 5.26 are the components of lift and drag that contribute to the total hand propulsive force. It is seen that hand propulsive force can be 100% from drag, 100% from lift, or somewhere in between. And although not all of these combinations of stroke angles and angles of attack are practical, this plot shows clearly again that there is more than one way to get down the pool. Similar plots were made for the arm alone (Fig. 5.27), and the arm and hand combined (Fig. 5.28). For the arm, Fig. 5.27 shows that drag totally dominates lift. For the hand and arm

combined, the optimum stroke angle that produces the most propulsive force is 0°, using an angle of attack of 90°—as before, straight backwards, with the palm facing directly toward the feet. Remember though, that there are several possible reasons why swimmers do not pull their arms exactly straight backwards, as described in the previous section.

It must be emphasized that all of these studies were for steady-state flow, where the direction, velocity, and orientation remained constant during the force evaluation. Neither the rotation of both the hand and arm together nor the relative rotation of the hand relative to the arm was evaluated. By rotating the palm so that it faces backwards sooner than the arm, propulsive force from the hand may begin sooner than it would have otherwise. Likewise, at the end

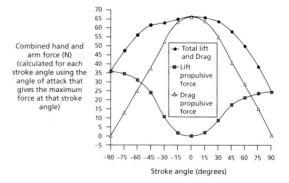

Fig. 5.28 Maximum hand and arm combined propulsive force vs. stroke angle. Velocity = 2 m · s^{-1}, turbulence intensity = 1%, turbulence length = 0.1 m.

of the stroke, swimmers keeping their hands facing backwards as long as possible during the upsweep might prolong the propulsion generated by the hand. However, when that hand begins decelerating, it is imperative for the swimmer to turn it sideways and get it out of the water as soon as possible. See the section on the effect of stroke acceleration and deceleration on propulsion.

Effect of hand and arm position on propulsion

Obviously, the position of the hand and arm during a stroke is very important. As an example, Fig. 5.29 shows three extremes of the many possible hand and arm positions during the freestyle. The position with the dropped elbow is a common position used by beginning swimmers that does not provide much propulsion. The straight arm position provides improved propulsion, but is not as efficient as the high-elbow position for two reasons:

1 The large moment associated with the straight arm pull requires more energy to move the arm through the water than if the arm were moving closer to the body, as with the high-elbow pull. *A moment is a force times a distance.* In this case, the moment is the propulsive force of the hand and arm multiplied by the distance from the shoulder to where the force is acting. When the arm is closer to the shoulder this distance is less, the moment is less, and less energy is expended. As an example, hold some barbells in both hands at your side. The weight you are supporting is the weight of the barbells. The force is downward, and there is little moment associated with supporting the weight, because the line of action of the force passes close to the shoulder. Continue holding the barbells, but now rotate your arms up, keeping them straight, until they are horizontal and in front of you. You are still supporting the weight of the barbells, but now there is also a moment which is equal to the weight of the barbells times the distance from the shoulder to the barbells. It takes a lot more energy to hold the barbells in this position.

2 The straight arm position does not employ the strong back muscles as effectively as does the high-elbow position.

It is also beneficial during the *recovery* part of a stroke to keep the elbow high and close in to the head. This

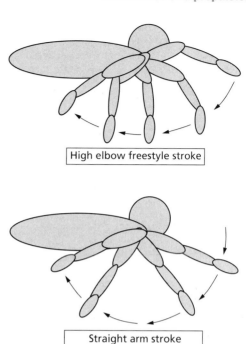

High elbow freestyle stroke

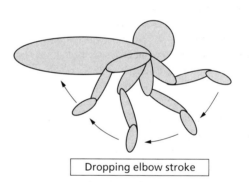

Straight arm stroke

Dropping elbow stroke

Fig. 5.29 Three extremes of hand and arm positions in the freestyle.

lessens the moment during the recovery process, and again requires less energy than if the arm were held straight during a wide recovery.

Another way in which position can affect propulsion is the location of the hand and arm relative to other parts of the body or the water surface. Interference drag comes into play when the hand or arm gets close to the torso (freestyle, butterfly) or head (backstroke, breaststroke). Wave drag must be considered at any point in a stroke cycle where the hand or arms are near the surface. These effects are, however, difficult to quantify since no research has been done in this area.

Effect of hand and arm velocity on propulsion

Within the range of hand and arm velocities that result in significant propulsive forces, the boundary layer is turbulent. Assuming that wave and interference drag are not active, from strictly a mechanical perspective, higher stroke velocities are always better, unless by starting a stroke too fast, a swimmer cannot continue to accelerate throughout the stroke (see next subsection).

Effect of stroke acceleration and deceleration on propulsion

The effects of acceleration and deceleration have been investigated by Thayer (1990), Sanders (1999), and Riewald and Bixler (2001a, 2001b). All of them showed that acceleration (or deceleration) plays a significant role in propulsion. By accelerating their arms and hands, swimmers can greatly increase the propulsive force they are generating.

Thayer conducted sophisticated experimental tests with a hand model in a flume, and included rotation as well as translation in the test. She found that the unsteady flow affected drag more than it did lift. Thayer also determined that the unsteady effects caused by arm rotation increased drag force beyond that of steady drag force by amounts between 5 and 15 N during the stroke.

Sanders conducted tests in a tow tank for steady flow and for the hand accelerating from 0.0 to $0.6\,\text{m}\cdot\text{s}^{-1}$ for accelerations ranging up to $7\,\text{m}\cdot\text{s}^{-2}$. Only the effects of acceleration in the direction of the flow were included. Sander's model was submerged to avoid wave drag on the hand. And although he subtracted the drag of the hand support alone from the drag of the hand with the support, interference drag between the hand support and hand itself was not accounted for. Sanders steady-state coefficients were smaller than those found by Schleihauf, Berger, Riewald, and Thayer, and it is not clear why his results are different. Even so, his results on a relative basis also showed that acceleration can have a significant effect on propulsive forces. Also, since his test setup eliminated wave drag and ventilation, the axial component of force on the hand was allowed to fully develop, and, like Riewald, he found the axial forces to be significant.

Riewald's study, using CFD, determined that swimmers can actually create a negative propulsive force if they decelerate their hand and arm too quickly, even though they still may be moving their hand and arm backwards relative to the water. The results of this study were discussed earlier, where the acceleration effects were correlated with the acceleration number. Like Bixler's study for steady flow (Bixler 2002), Riewald investigated which combination of stroke angle and angle of attack provided the most propulsive forward force, and again, the optimum direction to stroke was found to be directly backwards with the hand held at an angle of attack of $90°$ (palm facing the feet). Two other facts from the CFD analyses are worth mentioning:

1 In agreement with Thayer's results, drag and axial forces are affected by acceleration and deceleration more than lift forces are affected. So, in an ideal world, if it were practical, swimmers should stroke in a direction to maximize propulsive drag during acceleration phases of their stroke, and if and when they must decelerate their hands and arms, they should rotate them so that they are using mainly lift propulsion.

2 Second, swimmers should not just focus on hand propulsion. The arm plays a more important part than steady-state analysis would indicate during drag-dominant propulsion. For example, a hand and arm of $0.12\,\text{m}$ width and accelerating from 0.5 to $2.0\,\text{m}\cdot\text{s}^{-1}$ in $0.25\,\text{s}$ ($6\,\text{m}\cdot\text{s}^{-2}$) has an acceleration number of 0.46. Using Riewald's results, at this acceleration number the drag force for the hand is 1.55 times that predicted by the quasi-steady technique, while the arm drag is more than 2.1 times that predicted by the quasi-steady technique. The probable reason why the arm is affected more by acceleration than the hand is that there is room on the more gradually curved arm surface for the separation line of the boundary layer to shift along the surface and change the pressure profile on the surface. The hand edge is much sharper, and no significant movement of the boundary layer separation point can take place.

One of the advantages of the CFD method (Riewald & Bixler 2001a, 2001b) over most experimental techniques is the ability to easily visualize the flow with a variety of graphical techniques. A method used in wind tunnels to visualize the flow patterns on the surface of an object is called the oil film technique. Using this method, oil with a small amount of fluorescent

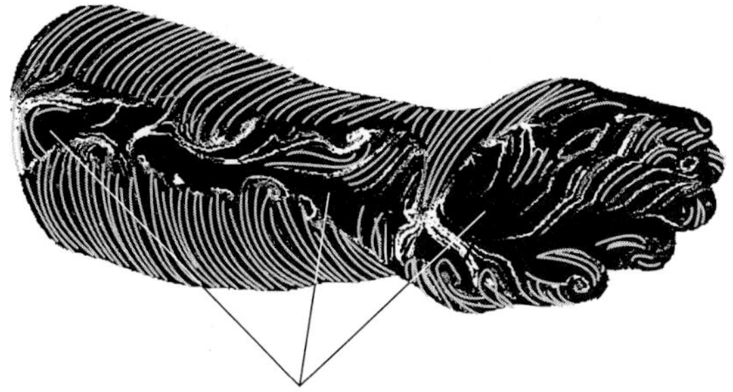

'Cleared' areas show where the
boundary layer has separated

Fig. 5.30 CFD oil film plot shows the boundary layer separation on the downstream side of a swimmer's hand and arm.

dye is applied to the surface of the object. The oil flows slowly during the test, and the direction of motion is picked up under fluorescent lighting. The same thing may be performed "analytically," using a CFD model. The oil film plot shown in Fig. 5.30 shows clearly on the downstream side of the hand and arm where the boundary layer has separated. Contour plots of many different variables, such as pressure, may also be created. General pathlines of flow may also be plotted through the fluid domain, showing the direction of the fluid flow as illustrated in Fig. 5.10. Counsilman (1968) deduced that the "price of acceleration is costly" (in terms of energy). From the CFD study we now know that the price of deceleration is also costly (in terms of negative propulsion).

Summary of hand and arm propulsion

On the basis of the results that have been presented herein, there are a few basics concerning hand and arm propulsion that should be emphasized:
• The arm plays an important role in propulsion
• Regardless of the stroke angle at which the arm is moving, keep the palm of the hand facing directly toward the feet to maximize propulsion.
• There are many combinations of stroke angle and angle of attack that provide propulsive components from both drag and lift forces. A combination that results in equal lift and drag forces provides almost as much propulsive force as a combination that provides a propulsive force that is based upon 100% drag (arm moves straight backwards). However, there are

several reasons (finding still water, balancing the body, lengthening the stroke) why a straight backstroke may not be desirable.
• Acceleration is good—it magnifies the propulsive force. Deceleration is bad—it can actually result in negative propulsion even though the hand and arm are still moving backwards. If you are "dead" at the end of a race, reduce the starting velocity of your stroke to the point where you can maintain accelerated motion through most of the stroke.

Foot and leg propulsion

When it comes to propulsion research, the legs and feet have not received nearly the attention accorded to the hands. Certainly much of this derives from the fact that the hands generate most of the propulsion. Still, there are some unique aspects concerning foot propulsion that are worth exploring.

The three types of kicks used in competitive swimming are the dolphin kick, the breaststroke kick, and the flutter kick (which is used in both the freestyle and the backstroke). There are many variations to these kicks, especially the flutter kick (straight 2-beat, crossover 2-beat, 6-beat, etc.). We will not get into the details of each type of kick, but will discuss the general characteristics of each of the three kicks.

Kicks provide propulsion and help swimmers to keep their bodies aligned in the right direction as they stroke and roll their bodies from side to side. In other words, they act as stabilizers, especially in the freestyle and backstroke, where the stroke motion is not symmetric about the long axis of the body. They perform a function similar to that of a sailboat keel. For without a keel, a fast sailboat would roll right over, much like what happens to my dog—a Welsh Corgi with a long body and very short legs—when she gets into a swimming pool. She easily loses her balance while trying to swim, and rolls over as easily as a log.

Whether or not the legs and feet offer *significant* propulsion is a question that often arises. A related question, assuming that the legs *can* contribute to propulsion, is whether they *should* be used for propulsion. Perhaps the energy expended to move the large leg muscles would be better spent on the arm strokes, which are the primary source of propulsion.

Obviously, legs do offer some propulsive capability when they are used alone—witness the kick sets that swimmers perform with their arms fixed on kickboards. But the speeds involved there are much slower than those of race speeds. The question really is, can swimmers push the water backwards with their feet faster than the arms are pulling the body through the water while at race speeds. If not, then the feet are not contributing to the propulsion at race speeds.

The flutter kick

Counsilman (1968) investigated the propulsive effectiveness of the flutter kick. He set up a tow test of swimmers and measured the tension in the towing rope when swimmers were kicking and when they were just being towed in a streamlined position. The goal was to see if the tension in the tow line while a swimmer was kicking was greater, less, or the same as when a swimmer was not kicking. He found that most swimmers' kicks became ineffective (as indicated by a tension equal to that of being towed in a streamlined position) between velocities of 1.3 and 1.5 m · s^{-1}, and in fact, in some instances, the drag actually increased for speeds above 1.5 m · s^{-1}. Below 1.3 m · s^{-1}, kicking increased propulsion, as indicated by a reduced tension in the tow line.

Taking this fact by itself, one might conclude that kicking is a waste of time in the sprints. However, countering this argument is that sprinters, by kicking, keep their legs from dropping lower into the water. Such a drop would increase the swimmer's form drag. It may be that swimmers' legs, when being towed, take up a different position than during regular swimming. Another possible conclusion is that the slower distance swimmers can increase their propulsion by kicking hard. However, from an energy standpoint, this is not practical in a long race.

So where does that leave us? Another useful study summarized by Counsilman (1968) compares the energy cost of swimming (as measured by required oxygen) with legs only, arms only, and with both together. The results show that above a velocity of 0.95 m · s^{-1}, it takes more energy to swim with the arms only, while below 0.95 m · s^{-1}, it takes more energy to swim with the arms stroking and the legs kicking. This would seem to imply that kicking legs are indeed useful in keeping the body horizontal in the water, especially for the sprints.

Probably the most useful study was one performed by Hollander *et al.* (1988), where using the MAD system (discussed earlier), they measured forces for swimmers moving with and without kicking and confirmed that kicking did indeed improve performance.

The dolphin kick

The dolphin kick, so-called because the legs move together like the fluke of a dolphin, goes with the butterfly stroke. There are two kick cycles for each arm stroke cycle. The timing of the kicks relative to the arm motions is critical. It should be noted that when butterflyers are swimming on the surface, not only do their legs oscillate, but also their upper bodies (especially women). However, below the surface, the oscillation is mostly limited to the legs. Various aspects of both types of oscillations will be addressed in the present section as well as the following section on body motion.

The Strouhal number (S) was introduced in Chapter 4 as a dimensionless parameter that is important when there is some type of frequency associated with fluid flow. It was defined as

$$S = nL/V \qquad (5.16)$$

where n is the frequency of the cyclic condition (cycles · s^{-1}), L is the characteristic length (m), and V is the velocity (m · s^{-1})

The Strouhal number is a useful parameter for characterizing the motion of a butterfly swimmer, where the characteristic length could be either the height of the swimmer or the width of the wake created by the shedding of vortices from the swimmer's feet. V is the average velocity of the swimmer, and n is the rate (cycles · s^{-1} or Hz) at which the swimmer kicks.

As an example, let us calculate the Strouhal number for an elite swimmer. If we are interested in the whole body motion along the surface, then we will use the swimmer's height as the characteristic length. Assume the swimmer is 1.75 m tall and moves at an average velocity of 1.9 m · s^{-1} and takes 1.2 s to complete each arm stroke cycle. This means that a single kick cycle would take 0.6 s (assuming that each kick takes the same amount of time). Therefore the

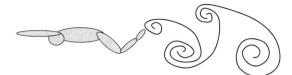

Fig. 5.31 Typical wake behind an underwater butterfly kick.

frequency n would be 1 cycle per 0.6 s or 1.67 cycles · s^{-1}. The Strouhal number based upon length would be $(1.67)(1.75)/1.9 = 1.54$.

Now let us examine the same swimmer, but turn our interest to butterfly kicking beneath the surface (where it is mainly the legs that are moving). In this case a better parameter for characteristic length would be the width of the wake created by the vortices shed from the swimmer's feet. There has been research examining the wakes of swimmers, especially for the butterfly kick. Persyn and Colman (1997) released dye from the feet of a swimmer doing the butterfly kick, allowing for a clear visualization of the wake behind the swimmer. Other studies by Arellano (Arellano 1999; Arellano *et al.* 2002), where bubbles were released from the feet, show that the wake width begins at approximately 1 m, but by the time the swimmer makes two more kick cycles, it expands to almost 1.5 m. If we use 1.5 as the characteristic length, then the Strouhal number of the swimmer discussed previously becomes $1.67(1.5)/1.9 = 1.32$. A typical wake geometry from these studies and others is shown in Fig. 5.31, where the wake is seen to be composed of vortices, shed alternatively from one side and then the other, behind the swimmer's feet. Note that the upper vortex, created by the weaker upward kick, is smaller than the lower vortex, created by the stronger downward kick.

It is now of interest to compare this wake geometry and Strouhal number with that of an aquatic propulsive system that utilizes oscillating airfoils to generate thrust. It has been known since the 1930s that thrust could be generated by an oscillating foil. That theory has been confirmed by many studies, including one by Triantafyllou *et al.* (1991) who determined that the *optimum* propulsive efficiency for such a system occurred at Strouhal numbers of between 0.25 and 0.35. For his evaluation, Triantafyllou used the width of the airfoil's wake for the characteristic length.

Table 5.4 Minimum and maximum Strouhal numbers of fish and cetaceans swimming at or near their maximum observed speed.

Fish or cetacean	Strouhal number	
	Minimum	Maximum
Bonito	0.27	0.33
Goldfish	0.28	0.31
Dolphin	0.29	0.31
Bream	0.31	0.33
Salmon	0.18	0.32
Bluefish	0.34	0.36
Cod	0.25	0.35
Shark	0.25	0.27
Jack mackerel	0.27	0.33
Rainbow trout	0.25	0.38

With the assistance of Woods Hole Oceanographic Institute, Triantafyllou then tabulated the Strouhal numbers of a wide variety of fish, ranging from goldfish to sharks, as well as dolphins. Using the width of the wake behind the fish for the characteristic length, he determined that all of them swung their tails with a frequency that gave them a Strouhal number between 0.2 and 0.4—exactly in the range where the airfoil propulsive efficiency was optimum (Table 5.4). A typical vortex trail behind a fish is shown in Fig. 5.32.

Thus, it appears that the optimum propulsion developed from either man-made or animal kicking motions is achieved with a Strouhal number of approximately 0.3. This is quite different from the 1.3 Strouhal number achieved by swimmers.

Sometimes you may hear an "expert" talk about swimming like a fish. Let us quantify what this means in terms of the butterfly kick. Using the

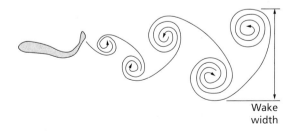

Fig. 5.32 Typical wake behind a swimming fish.

aforementioned example, an elite butterflyer might have a Strouhal number of 1.32 with the following components: $n = 1.67$ cycles$\cdot$s^{-1}, wake width $= 1.5$ m, and velocity $= 1.9$ m $\cdot$ s^{-1}. To swim like a fish, the butterflyer would need to get the Strouhal number down to about 0.3. This can be accomplished by changing any or all of the three components that make up the Strouhal number. If we just changed the velocity, and left the wake wide and kick frequency constant, the velocity would have to increase to 8.35 m $\cdot$ s^{-1}! If we just changed the kick frequency, it would have to be reduced to 0.38 cycles $\cdot$ s^{-1}, which means that each kick cycle would take 2.63 s and each arm stroke would take longer than 5.3 s! Finally, if we kept the frequency and velocity the same and changed the wake width, the wake width would be reduced to 0.34 m, which corresponds roughly to the feet themselves traveling only $+0.09$ m about the axis of the swimmer. None of these scenarios is even close to realistic, nor is any combination of changes. We humans were not designed like fish, so the next time someone suggests that you swim like a fish, ask them about the Strouhal number.

Having said all that, it is still worth studying how fish propel themselves, for although we humans were not designed to swim as efficiently as fish, we may indeed, albeit clumsily, use some of the same propulsive techniques. There is an abundance of research that has been done on the mechanics of swimming fish, and it is embarrassingly sophisticated compared to any of the research that has been done for swimmers. Several papers for suggested reading are included in the references, including some by Frank E. Fish (1993, 1998), a well-known and appropriately named expert in the field. Other well-known references on the precise creation and shedding of vortices in relation to aquatic animal propulsion are the classic works of Gray (1968), Lighthill (1975), Wu (1971), Wu et al. (1975), and Childress (1981).

Figures 5.31 and 5.32 show that the wakes behind a fish and a swimmer doing the butterfly kick are similar. The mechanism for fish propulsion is thought to work as follows: The fish tail swishes outward, forming a vortex, then quickly the tail swishes back in the reverse direction, producing another vortex. The second vortex rotates in the opposite direction from the first. The two vortices meet, momentum is transferred, and thrust is generated, either by the first vortex being canceled out by the second, or by the creation of

a propulsive jet from the combination of the two vortices. This jet results in a strong forward thrust as well as a lesser lateral thrust. This is a bit of a simplification, but it captures the essence of how the propulsion occurs. Readers interested in additional comparisons between dolphins and human swimmers are referred to Ungerechts et al. (1998). Ungerechts believes that if human swimmers emphasize the reverse action of their kicks, using a whip-like action, they are more likely to generate greater propulsion.

How much of the propulsion generated by a butterfly kick is from the proper creation and use of vortices is presently unknown. From Figs 5.31 and 5.32 we know that the wakes behind fish and swimmers can look somewhat the same. However, from the aforementioned calculations, we also know that a human Strouhal number is significantly different than those of dolphins or fish, making it likely that a significant portion of human propulsion does not come from vortex propulsion. Since the timing of the kicks, the locations of the vortices, and the speed of the swimmer must be exactly right for efficient vortex propulsion to occur, it is more likely that swimmers generate most of their propulsion from the butterfly kick in the same fashion that they generate propulsion with their legs in the flutter kick or with their hands and arms. That is, by moving their legs and feet through the water at certain angles and orientations, they create lift and drag forces, albeit not as large as those from the hands and arms. This is especially true for swimmers who can extend their feet to lie along the same axis of their legs or even beyond.

The breaststroke kick

The breaststroke kick used by most swimmers today involves a diagonal sweep of the legs through the water, where the soles of the feet are the primary propulsive surfaces. Because of the orientations and angles that swimmers must place their legs and feet in to obtain the best propulsion, flexibility of the joints is very important. There may also be some truth to the opinion that genetics (the structure of one's legs and feet) can also play a role in who becomes a good breaststroker. They are often said to "walk like a duck." Since a swimmer will accelerate and decelerate more in the breaststroke than in the other strokes, the timing of the arms and feet is critical. Maglischo (2003) provides an excellent discussion of all the nuances involved with this sometimes difficult stroke.

There are many unique points to the breaststroke, but one not often discussed is the interaction of breast-strokers' legs with their own internal waves. In the freestyle, backstroke, and butterfly, swimmers will generate waves (internal wave drag) that continually emanate from their bodies, and spread out beside and behind them. They have no "further" interaction with those waves unless it is at the ends of the pool when they execute their turns. In the breaststroke, there are large differences in velocity at different points during a stroke cycle. Thus, it becomes possible for a trailing transverse wave (see wave drag) moving at roughly the same average velocity of the swimmer to actually "catch up" with the swimmer temporarily during a slow point in the cycle. This will possibly increase the pressure loading on the legs or even torsos of the swimmers, in effect, giving a little extra pressure "push" from behind. A more obvious demonstration of this phenomenon occurs when a fast-moving boat, approaching a dock, slows down. The trailing transverse wave will catch up to the boat and as it moves ahead of the boat, will give it a bit of forward motion.

Body motion and position

There are hundreds of things you should not do with your body. The ones that concern swimming are listed below. They all result in increased resistive drag or reduced propulsive drag.
- Excessive up and down motion
- Excessive lateral motion
- Horizontal and vertical body misalignment
- Bad streamlines such as hands not fully clasped, head up, legs dragging, etc.
- Breathing techniques such as a slight lifting of the head rather then just turning it to the side.
- Static body position in the water (little body rotation)

It has been suggested that perhaps, in the breast-stroke and butterfly, swimmers can actually get some additional propulsion by the undulation of their bodies, where water is accelerated backwards by a "body wave" that travels toward their feet. Many

investigations have explored this possibility, but probably the most meaningful study for the butterfly was conducted by Sanders et al. (1995). Fourier analyses were made to determine the frequency, amplitude, and phase characteristics of the vertical undulation of the head vertex, shoulders, hips, knees, and ankles. There was a strong relationship between the velocities of the first Fourier frequency wave and the center of mass, suggesting that indeed the body was contributing to a propulsive "whip-like" action. However, unlike the butterfly study, a similar one done for the breast-stroke by Sanders et al. (1998) found that the body wave is probably not propulsive.

Water entry

Water entry refers to the piercing of the water surface by the hands, head, arms, or any other body part, including the start from the blocks. Wave and splash drag are associated with water entry, and the more splash you see when a swimmer enters the water, the larger is the drag associated with entry.

There has been a tremendous amount of research concerning water entry that has been financed by the military establishments of various countries around the world. Some of it is now unclassified, but unfortunately, usually the sizes and velocities involved are too large to provide information of use to swimmers. The best rule of thumb is an old one: try to put all parts of your body "through the same hole" in the water. Doing this results in less splash, and hence less drag upon entry.

Swimming theories

There have been several "theories," related to swimmer propulsion. Human nature, being what it is, compels us to create new buzzwords or theories to describe old phenomena. This happens in every human field of endeavor. For example, in the business world, by developing a program of "Continuous Improvement" or "Total Quality" and adding in some new tools and buzzwords, we feel we are making progress (as opposed to just saying that we are going to work harder and smarter). So it is with swimming propulsion theories. We have the weaving back theory, the paddle theory, the Bernoulli theory, and the vortex theory. In fact, no matter how you move your hands and feet, and no matter what you call it, it all gets back to Newton's laws of motion. Whether you weave your hands in the water or pull straight back, it is Newton that will get you to the wall. Although many still cling to the Bernoulli theory of propulsion, it has been shown without question that it does not apply to swimming. Newton is the man. Even the vortex theory, which involves transfer of momentum from one vortex to another, is dependent upon Sir Isacc.

So, having already covered Newton's laws, this author would prefer to ignore the buzzwords and move on. However, in good conscience this will not be done because (1) some of the theories help to emphasize certain concepts previously presented, and (2) some of the theories need exposure as to how, or even if, they apply to swimming.

Propulsive drag theories focused on how to move the hands and arms (straight back, s-shaped pull, etc.). The leader in their developments was J.E. Counsilman (1968). These were followed by the propulsive lift theory wherein the application of Bernoulli's principle was presented as the explanation of the lift generated by swimmers. Counsilman (1971), always looking for a better understanding of swimming, also led the way with Bernoulli. Since then, it has been shown experimentally by Ferrell (1991) and analytically by Bixler (1999) that (1) Counsilman was correct in determining that swimmers use lift as well as drag to create propulsive force, and (2) that the lift generated by swimmers' hands is not correctly described by Bernoulli's principle. This is because Bernoulli's principle applies only to ideal flow where the flow remains attached to the surface, and both Ferrel and Bixler showed that the boundary layer separates from the surface of the hand. Even now, there are still those who insist on invoking Bernoulli's principle because of the misconception that lift is the type of force generated only by airplane wings, whereas in reality, lift is merely a force that is perpendicular to the drag force, no matter how it was developed.

Colwin (1984) has attempted, using airfoil lift theory, to explain how swimmers generate predominantly lift-force propulsion based upon a vortex system composed of a starting vortex, a bound vortex, and a trailing or finishing vortex. Simple airfoil lift theory is based upon inviscid flow, and involves "circulation" of flow around the airfoil. The vortex theory suggests that lift-force propulsion is developed in unsteady flow primarily by the directional changes of a foil-shaped hand as it moves through the stroke and sets up the mechanics necessary for creating flow circulation. This theory requires that swimmers be skilled and dexterous enough to establish and control the necessary flow circulation and propel themselves forward through the rapid generation and shedding of vortices.

It would be wonderful indeed if we humans had such control, but there are several reasons why this theory is not valid:

1 It is one thing to control the flow on a nice smooth airfoil, but the human hand is a different story. An airfoil and hand are aerodynamically very different, as shown by the polar plots of lift vs. drag for a low aspect ratio airfoil and a human hand (Fig. 5.24).

2 The flow circulation airfoil lift theory and accompanying vortex system exist only for inviscid flow conditions with no boundary layer separation. One exception is that viscosity must be temporarily taken into account to explain the formation of the starting vortex, but after that, the calculation of lift based upon circulation is done using the laws of inviscid flow. The research of Ferrel (1991) and Bixler (1999), both discussed previously, has shown that even for low velocities and low angles of attack, the flow is viscous, with significant boundary layer separation (Fig. 5.10). This holds true for either steady or unsteady flow. In fact, even for simple airfoils, above about a 15° angle of attack, separated flow occurs.

3 The center of mass velocity patterns for swimmers indicate that swimmers actually decelerate as they make changes in hand and arm speed and direction (Maglischo 2003), and usually accelerate to peak velocity during the middle of each propulsive phase of their underwater armstrokes.

Readers interested in an accurate description of airfoil lift theory are referred to Schlichting and Truckenbrodt (1979) or any other introductory book on aerodynamics. However, readers interested in swimming propulsion would be better served by a quick review of Newton's laws of motion.

Swimming mechanics: where should we go from here?

We MUST improve our tools to evaluate the mechanics of swimming. Here are a few suggestions on where, outside of our little swimming box, we should look to do that.

• We should seek out the testing and analysis expertise of technical experts in mainstream engineering fields such as aerodynamics, fluid dynamics, and naval architecture. These people have many tools and techniques, both analytical and experimental that could greatly enhance our knowledge of swimming. Computational fluid dynamics (CFD) is one example of such a tool. There are *many, many* others.

• We should study the results of past research in fields that are applicable to swimming. The incompressible flow research performed by aerodynamicists in the 1930s is one example. Why has no one looked at this area? The unsteady flow research done in the eighteenth and nineteenth centuries is another example. It is astonishing that we have not used technology that has been around since the late 1700s and early 1800s.

• Researchers in the mechanics of animal swimming have a mathematical prowess far surpassing what has been demonstrated by most human swimming scientists. These capabilities have allowed them to advance their knowledge about animal swimming well beyond what we know about humans. Let us improve our math understanding so we can use more advanced mathematical techniques.

It is hoped that we can advance the state-of-the-art in swimming mechanics. In doing so, we will make ourselves less vulnerable to believing every new fad and every new buzzword that comes along.

References

Arellano, R. (1999) Vortices and propulsion. In: R. Sanders & J. Linsten, eds. *XVII International Symposion on Biomechanics in Sports*. Perth, Australia: Western Australia School of Biomedical and Spovgcrts Sciences, pp. 53–66.

Arellano, R., Pardillo, S. & Gavilan, A. (2002) Underwater undulatory swimming kinematic characteristics, vortex generation and application during start, turn, and swimming strokes. *XX International Symposium on Biomechanics in Sports,* Caceres, Spain.

Berger, M., de Groot, G. & Hollander, A. (1995) Hydrodynamic drag and lift forces on human hand/arm models. *Journal of Biomechanics* **2**, 125–133.

Bixler, B. (1999) The computational fluid dynamics of a swimmer's hand and arm. Report to USA Swimming.

Bixler, B. (2004). The Fastskin II Swimsuit. Fluent CFD Summit Conference, Dearborn, Michigan.

Bixler, B. & Riewald, S. (2002) Analysis of a swimmer's hand and arm in steady flow conditions using computational fluid dynamics. *Journal of Biomechanics* **35**, 713–717.

Blasius, H. (1908) Grenzschichten in Flüssigkeiten mit kleiner Reiburg. *Zeitschrift für Mathematik und Physik* **56**, 1–37.

Childress, S. (1981) *Mechanics of Swimming and Flying*. Cambridge, UK: Cambridge University Press.

Colwin, C. (1984) Fluid dynamics: vortex circulation in swimming propulsion. In: T.F. Welsh, ed. *ASCA World Clinic Yearbook*. Ft Lauderdale, FL: American Swimming Coaches Association, pp. 38–46.

Counsilman, J. (1968) *The Science of Swimming*. Englewood Cliffs, NJ: Prentice-Hall.

di Prampero, P., Pendergast, D., Wilson, D. & Rennie, D. (1974) Energetics of swimming man. *Journal of Applied Physiology* **37**, 1–5.

Efimov, Y., Chernin, K. & Shevalov, A. (1967) Calculation of the wave resistance of a thin ship in unsteady motion. *Tr. Leningrad Korablestroi Inst* **58**, 47–55.

Fage, A., Falkner, V.M. & Skan, S.W. (1929) Aeronautical Research Council Report No. 1241.

Ferrell, M. (1991) *An Analysis of the Bernoulli Lift Effect as a Propulsive Component of Swimming Strokes*. M.S. Thesis, State University of New York, College at Cortland.

Firby, H. (1975) *Howard Firby on Swimming*. London: Pelham Books.

Fish, F. (1993) Power output and propulsive efficiency of swimming bottlenose dolphins (*Tursiops truncatus*). *Journal of Experimental Biology* **185**, 179–193.

Fish, F. (1998) Comparative kinematics and hydrodynamics of odontocete cetaceans: morphological and ecological correlates with swimming performance. *Journal of Experimental Biology* **201**, 2867–2877.

Gray, J. (1968) *Animal Locomotion*. London: Weidenfeld and Nicolson.

Hay, J. & Thayer, A. (1989) Flow visualization of competitive swimming techniques: the tufts method. *Journal of Biomechanics* **22**(1), 11–19.

Hoerner, S.F. (1965) *Fluid Dynamic Drag*. Brick Town, NJ: S.F. Hoerner.

Hollander, A., de Groot, G., van Ingen Schneau, G., Kahman, R. & Toussaint, H. (1988) Contributions of the legs to propulsion in front crawl swimming. In:

B. Ungerechts, K. Wilkie & K. Reischle, eds. *International Series on Sport Sciences, Vol. 18: Swimming Science V*. Champaign, IL: Human Kinetics, pp. 39–43, 69.

Ikegami, K. & Imaizumi, Y. (1979) Prediction and model experiments on speed loss of a ship in waves. Mitsuibishi Technical Bulletin No. 137.

Iversen, H. & Balent, R. (1951). A correlating modulus for fluid resistance in accelerated motion. *Journal of Applied Physics* **22**(3), 324–328.

Kelvin, Lord (1887) Ship Waves. Trans. IME, London.

Keys, C. & Wiesner, R. (1975) Guidelines for reducing helicopter parasite drag. *Journal of the American Helicopter Society* **20** (1).

Kolmogorov, S. & Duplisheheva, A. (1992) Active drag, useful mechanical power output and hydrodynamic force coefficient in different swimming strokes at maximal velocity. *Journal of Biomechanics* **25**, 311–318.

Lighthill, J. (1975) *Mathematical Biofluiddynamics*. Philadelphia: Society for Industrial and Applied Mathematics.

Liu, C., Kline, S. & Johnston, J. (1966) An experimental study of turbulent boundary layer on rough walls. Report MD-15. Thermosciences Division, Department of Mechanical Engineering, Stanford University.

Lyttle, A. & Blanksby, B. (2000) A look at gliding and underwater kicking in the swim turn. In: *ISBS 2000, Applied Proceedings of the XVIII International Symposium on Biomechanics in Sports*, Hong Kong.

Maglischo, E.W. (2003) *Swimming Fastest*. Champaign, IL: Human Kinetics.

Persyn, U. & Colman, V. (1997) Flow visualization and propulsion in undulated swimming techniques. *Tecnicas simultaneas e ondulatorias: desafios contemporaneos em natacao*, Porto.

Riewald, S. & Bixler, B. (2001a) Computation of lift and drag forces for a model of a swimmer's hand and arm in unsteady flow using computational fluid dynamics. Report for the USOC Sport Science and Technology Committee.

Riewald, S. & Bixler, B. (2001b) CFD Analysis of a swimmer's arm and hand acceleration and deceleration. In: J. Blackwell, ed. *XIX International Symposium on Biomechanics in Sports*. San Francisco: University of San Francisco, pp 117–119.

Rom, J. (1992) *High Angle of Attack Aerodynamics—Subsonic, Transonic, and Supersonic Flows*. New York: Springer-Verlag.

Rota, J. (1962) Turbulent boundary layers in incompressible flow. *Progress in Aero Sciences, Vol. 2*. Oxford, UK: Pergamon Press, pp. 1–219.

Sanders, R. (1999) Hydrodynamic characteristics of a swimmer's hand. *Journal of Applied Biomechanics* **15**, 3–26.

Sanders, R., Cappaert, J. & Devlin, R. (1995) Wave characteristics of butterfly swimming. *Journal of Biomechanics* **28**, 9–16.

Sanders, R., Cappaert, J. & Pease, D. (1998) Wave characteristics of Olympic breaststroke swimmers. *Journal of Applied Biomechanics* **14**, 40–51.

Schleihauf, R. (1979) A hydrodynamic analysis of swimming propulsion. In: J. Terauds & E.W. Bedingfield, eds. *International Series on Sport Sciences, Vol. 8: Swimming III*. Baltimore, MD: University Park Press, pp. 70–110.

Schemensky, R. (1973) Development of an empirically based computer program to predict the aerodynamic characteristics of aircraft. AFFDL-TR-73-144, Vols. I and II.

Schlichting, O. (1934) Ship resistance in water of limited depth. *Jahrbuch der STG* **35**.

Schlichting, H. (1987) *Boundary Layer Theory*. New York: McGraw-Hill.

Schlichting, H. & Truckenbrodt, E. (1979) *Aerodynamics of the Airplane*. New York: McGraw-Hill International.

Sharp, R. & Costill, D. (1989) Influence of body hair removal physiological responses during breaststroke swimming. *Medicine and Science in Sports and Exercise* **21**(5), 576–580.

Takagi, H., Shimizu, Y., Kurashima, A. & Sanders, R. (2001) Effect of thumb abduction and adduction on hydrodynamic characteristics of a model of the human hand. *XIX International Symposium on Biomechanics in Sports*. San Francisco: University of San Francisco, pp. 122–126.

Thayer, A. (1990) *Hand Pressures as Predictors of Resultant and Propulsive Hand Forces in Swimming*. Ph.D. Dissertation. Iowa City, IA: University of Iowa.

Toussaint, H., de Groot, G., Savelberg, H., Vervoorn, K., Hollander, A. & van Ingern Schneau, G. (1988) Active drag related to velocity in male and female swimmers. *Journal of Biomechanics* **21**, 435–438.

Triantafyllou, M., Triantafyllou, G. & Gopalkrishnan, R. (1991) Wake mechanics for thrust generation in oscillating foils. *Physics of Fluids A* **12**, 2835–2837.

Troup, J. (1990) The effects of drafting on training and performance capacity. *International Center for Aquatics Research Annual*. Colorado Springs, CO, pp. 107–111.

Ungerechts, B., Daly, D. & Zhu, J. (1998) What dolphins tell us about hydrodynamics. *Journal of Swimming Research* **13**, 1–7.

Walsh, M. & Weinstein, L. (1978) Drag and heat transfer on surfaces with small longitudinal fins. In: *AIAA 11th Fluid Dynamics Conference*, Seattle, WA.

Wigley, C. (1931) Ship wave resistance. *Trans NECI* **47**.

Wigley, C. (1934) A comparison of experiment and calculated wave profiles and wave resistance for a form having parabolic waterlines. In: *Proceeding of the Royal Society*, London.

Wigley, C. (1962) The effect of viscosity on wave resistance. *Schiffstechnik Band* **9**.

Wood, T. (1977) *A Fluid Dynamic Analysis of the Propulsive Potential of the Hand and Forearm in Swimming*. M.S. Thesis. Halifax, Nova Scotia: Dalhousie University.

Wu, Y. (1971) Hydromechanics of swimming fishes and cetaceans. *Advances in Applied Mechanics* **11**, 1–63.

Wu, Y., Brokaw, C. & Brennen, C. (1975) *Swimming and Flying in Nature*. New York: Plenum Press.

Zdravkovich, M.M. & Pridden, D.L. (1977) Interference between two circular cylinders: series of unexpected discontinuities. *Journal of Industrial Aerodynamics* **2**, 255–270.

Recommended reading

Fox, R.W. & McDonald, A.T. (1992) *Introduction to Fluid Mechanics*. New York: John Wiley & Sons.

Schlichting, H. & Gersten, K. (2000) *Boundary-Layer Theory*, 8th edn. New York: Springer-Verlag.

Chapter 6
Psychology

John S. Raglin and Brendon S. Hale

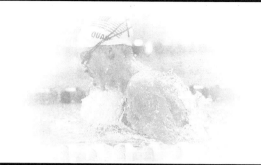

Introduction

The belief that psychology plays a role in swimming and other sports is not new. Over 100 years ago Dudley (1888) stated that "in all success in athletics the mental qualities of the athlete figure largely" (p. 43.). However, just as in the case of the contribution of physiological factors to sport performance, the influence of psychology in sport is complex. It has been recognized that an array of variables can come into play before, during, and after sport events, including both relatively stable factors, such as personality traits, as well as more transient psychological states that may change from moment to moment. These variables may act independently or interact with one another to either improve or harm performance. Additionally, the specific effect of a given psychological factor may well depend upon the type of sport or the skill level of an athlete.

Among psychological variables, the personality of the athlete has been among the earliest topics of study in the field of sport psychology, and unfortunately, the results of this research have resulted in unnecessary contradiction and confusion regarding the role that personality plays in sport success. One reason for this confusion stems from the fact that unlike other fields of study in exercise science, sport psychology deals with concepts that are common to human experience. Unlike concepts such as muscle morphology or somatotype, virtually everyone has some degree of understanding of psychological concepts such as personality, stress, and anxiety. Unfortunately lay definitions

of these and other psychological variables may vary considerably from person to person, and are often inconsistent with their use within academia. Hence, in the following sections on psychology, an effort is made to define crucial terminology in accordance with generally accepted definitions.

Predisposing psychological factors in sport performance: personality

Personality has been defined as "relatively enduring differences among people in specifiable tendencies to perceive the world in a certain way and in dispositions to react or behave in a specified manner with predictable regularity" (Spielberger, Gorsuch & Luschene 1983, p. 1). Personality traits are most commonly assessed using so-called pencil and paper questionnaires, and a variety of validated measures of personality have been developed and successfully employed in both general psychology and sport psychology research. Additionally, a large number of personality and other psychological measures have been developed specifically for athletes (Ostrow 1990). Although it has been proposed that these sport-specific measures are more useful for research and provide greater application in sport settings, this contention has not been consistently borne out from the findings of experimental studies with athletes and there is no compelling evidence to support the use of psychological measures to select athletes for sport teams (Raglin 2001). A primary reason for this lack of effectiveness is that many of sport-specific psychological measures have not been developed using rigorously established procedures that ensure that the measures possess test validity (APA 1999), and this continues to be a problem in the field of sport psychology.

Early reviews of personality and athleticism research findings consistently indicated that athletes differed in personality structure from nonathletes in several dimensions. In particular it was found that successful athletes scored higher in measures of extroversion and emotional stability than less successful competitors and nonathletes (Warburton & Kane 1966; Cooper 1969). In contrast, reviews of the literature published the following decade drew a very different conclusion, and were nearly unanimous in declaring that the association between personality and sport performance was either minimal or altogether nonexistent (Rushall 1970; Martens 1975). As a result many sport psychologists abandoned the study of personality in athletes altogether.

These contradictory perspectives on the relative importance of personality were addressed in reviews by Morgan (1978a, 1980a), who concluded that much of the research that rejected the relationship between sport performance and personality suffered from serious methodological flaws. Among the problems noted by Morgan was the widespread failure to account for the potential occurrence of faked responses to psychological questionnaires, a phenomenon referred to as response distortion. There are a variety of ways in which individuals may distort their responses to psychological questionnaires and the most common is to "fake good" by invariantly responding to items in a stereotypically positive manner. The occurrence of response distortion can be detected through the use of "lie scales," but these measures have rarely been employed in sport psychology research. More carefully conducted research that accounted for the potential of response distortion was found to indicate that athletes did indeed possess unique personality traits, including above average scores for extroversion and emotional stability, and low scores in neuroticism and other measures of psychopathology (i.e., mental illness) and mood disturbance. These differences were generally small in magnitude and in many cases unsuccessful athletes were found to score only modestly better than the population norms of nonathletes for measures of emotional stability and neuroticism.

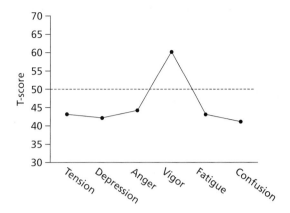

Fig. 6.1 Baseline Profile of Mood State (POMS) scores for a sample of college swimmers. Adapted from Raglin (1993).

On the basis of these findings and other research involving athletes in a variety of sports including swimming, Morgan (1978b, 1980b) developed a "mental health" model of sport performance. This model predicts that a negative relationship exists between psychopathology and sport performance, that is, athletes who are depressed, anxious, exhibit disturbed mood, or other forms of mental illness will perform more poorly than athletes who possess average or above average mental health. The prototypical mood state profile of successful athletes has come to be identified as the "iceberg profile" (see Fig. 6.1). Most elite athletes possess this profile the majority of the time, but it disappears during overtraining. The psychological characteristics associated with successful athletes have proven stable over time. Recent longitudinal research (Morgan & Costill 1996) with a sample of elite distance runners whose psychological profiles were contrasted across a span of 20 years revealed remarkably little change in their psychological characteristics, thus indicating that successful athletes continue to have better psychological health than unsuccessful athletes long after their competitive years.

Subsequent research by Morgan (1987, 1988) and other researchers has replicated this work with athletes in a variety of sports, skill levels and age groups, providing corroborating support for the efficacy of the mental health model (Mahoney 1989; Newcombe & Boyle 1995; LeUnes & Burger 2000).

Morgan (1985) later published a summary of research that examined the utility of the mental health model to accurately identify successful and unsuccessful athletes on the basis of psychological information. The studies involved samples of athletes in number of sports, including swimming, and skill level ranging from college to Olympic caliber. Using validated psychological measures developed in academic psychology, personality traits, mood state, and psychological states were assessed in collegiate and elite athletes and the resulting psychological profiles were contrasted between successful and unsuccessful competitors. In other studies, psychological profiles were used to make predictions about the future success or failure of athletes vying for positions on Olympic or international teams (Morgan & Johnson 1978). The results of these studies indicate that successful athletes generally possessed lower scores for such personality factors as introversion, depression, neuroticism, and trait anxiety. On the basis of psychological information alone, on average successful and unsuccessful athletes could be identified at an accuracy of ranging 70–85%, a rate higher than chance but clearly insufficient for the purpose of selecting athletes. Despite this apparent lack of practical application, the findings of mental health model research indicate that it is in the coach's best interest to consider not only the physical welfare of the athlete but also the athlete's mental health.

As measured by the POMS (Profile of Mood States) (McNair *et al.* 1992) the combination of low scores for undesirable or negative mood factors and a high score for the positive mood factor has been described as the "Iceberg Profile" (Morgan 1980a). Most elite athletes possess this profile the majority of the time, but it disappears during overtraining.

Selecting team members

The effectiveness of the mental health model in identifying successful and unsuccessful athletes has consistently exceeded chance levels of prediction. On average, from 70 to 85% of athletes could be correctly classified on the basis of psychological information. Despite this level of accuracy, Morgan (1985) cautioned against employing the mental health model in attempts to select athletes for competition. In virtually all mental health model research, some false classifications resulted. Cases in which athletes possess intermediate psychological scores preclude categorization as either successful or unsuccessful. Moreover, the level of accuracy achieved with mental health model studies is insufficient to select athletes, and there is no evidence that psychological identification models can be made more accurate (Eysenck *et al.* 1982; Vanden Auweele *et al.* 1993; Morgan 1997). Despite this, psychological measures have been and continue to be used to select athletes for professional sport teams (Smith 1997).

Training factors: mood state

Research has also shown that psychological variables in athletes may change in response to significant stressors. In a summary of 10 years of research with swimmers and other athletes, Morgan *et al.* (1987) found that mood was consistently associated with the current level of training athletes were undergoing. In each of these studies, mood was assessed by means of the POMS (McNair *et al.* 1992), a questionnaire that assesses the tension, depression, anger, vigor, fatigue, and confusion. In the majority of this research, these factors were combined to yield a single, general measure of total mood disturbance by subtracting the vigor score from the sum of the other factors and adding a constant of 100 to prevent negative values. Moods have been defined as subjective feelings that are more transient compared to personality traits that change little over a lifetime (McNair *et al.* 1992). Emotions such as anxiety may persist for a very brief period (e.g., a few seconds) and are often experienced with greater intensity than moods, which may last from minutes to weeks.

The results of studies of over 1000 swimmers and other athletes who underwent mood state monitoring during their training consistently revealed that changes in training volume are predictably related to alterations in mood disturbance season (Morgan *et al.* 1987; Raglin *et al.* 1991; Raglin & Morgan 1994). With increases in training distance there are corresponding elevations in mood disturbance and a reduction in the positive mood factor of vigor. Typically, the highest mood disturbance scores are observed at the peak of the training season. With reductions in training volume or tapers, mood disturbance falls in most athletes, and following the completion of the taper, mood scores generally return to values observed at the beginning of the training season. During the peak of training, mood scores on the negative POMS factors may equal or exceed population norms, reflecting a shift of 1–2 standard deviations. The mood state responses of men and women athletes undergoing comparable training have been found to be remarkably similar (Morgan *et al.* 1987; Raglin *et al.* 1991; Raglin & Morgan 1994), and recent research has replicated these findings with age group swimmers (Raglin *et al.* 2000). Figure 6.2 presents the typically observed relationship between training load and mood disturbance for a sample of college swimmers assessed across an entire training season.

Changes in specific POMS factors also exhibit this dose–response relationship, with the possible exception of tension. Raglin *et al.* (1991) found that POMS tension scores did not decrease during tapers in college swimmers, and it was speculated that this reflected the stress of conference championships to be held at the end of the season. In contrast, each of the other POMS factors responded positively to the reduction in training load. The failure for tension to fall during the taper may not be undesirable as other research indicates that between 30 and 45% athletes benefit from elevated anxiety (Hanin 1997).

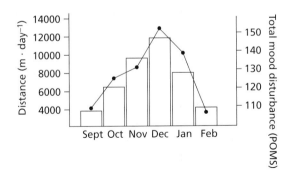

Fig. 6.2 Total mood state scores and average monthly training loads for a sample of swimmers assessed across a competitive season. Adapted from Raglin (1993).

Acute mood state responses to physical training

Not all physical conditioning regimens in swimming and other sports involve gradual adjustments to the training load that occur over weeks or months. For example, in the case of training camps, three- or fourfold increases in training volume may be rapidly imposed over periods as brief as a few days. Several mood state monitoring studies have been conducted to examine the psychological responses of swimmers undergoing such regimens. In these cases the administration of the POMS is modified in order to assess more acute or "state" aspects of mood state, and athletes complete the POMS or other psychological measures according to how they are feeling "today" or "right now."

O'Connor *et al.* (1991) observed the responses of collegiate men and women swimmers exposed to period of increased training from an average of 6800 m of swimming a day to 12 075 m across a 3-day period. Mood state was assessed using the "today" version of the POMS each morning, and daily measures were also taken of muscle soreness, perceived exertion, exercise heart rate to a paced swim, and salivary cortisol. It was found that elevations in mood disturbance occurred by the second day of increased training, and the responses were similar for both men and women swimmers. Significant elevations in perceived exertion (total and local) and muscle soreness also were observed, but salivary cortisol and exercise heart rate were unaffected by the increased training. These results suggest that mood state as measured by the POMS is a more sensitive indicator of the strain of acute physical training than commonly used physiological measures, a finding that has been replicated in work with distance runners (Verde *et al.* 1993).

A slightly longer training protocol was used in a study conducted by Morgan *et al.* (1988) to examine the responses of male collegiate swimmers to a 10-day period of intensified training. Unlike O'Connor *et al.* (1991) and the majority of monitoring research in which there is often some variation in the training load within the sample, both training volume and intensity were controlled. Each swimmer was prescribed a daily training load averaging 8900 m at a pace equaling 94% $\dot{V}_{O_{2max}}$. Mood state, muscle soreness,

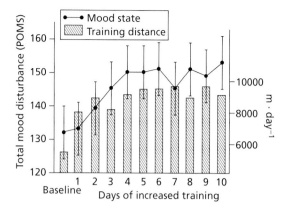

Fig. 6.3 Total mood state scores and daily training for a sample of college swimmers. Adapted from Morgan *et al.* (1988).

and perceived exertion were assessed daily, as were selected physiological variables (Costill *et al.* 1988). It was anticipated that some of the swimmers would have difficulty completing the training regimen (i.e., overreaching) and an attempt to identify such cases on the basis of the psychological and physiological information collected from the swimmers. A coach working with the swimmers made determinations of overreaching on the basis of difficulty in completing the training and elevated perception of training effort (double check details). Total mood disturbance scores for the group increased linearly in the entire sample during the initial 5 days of training before leveling off for the remainder of the training period. Similar trends were noted for perceived exertion and muscle soreness ratings, and the general trend for the entire sample is typified by the POMS results presented in Fig. 6.3.

Inspection of the individual data revealed that four swimmers exhibited pronounced elevations in their total mood scores. It was predicted that these individuals would have difficulty completing the training. Three swimmers were identified by the coach as showing signs of overreaching and each of these individuals were among the four identified on the basis of elevated mood state scores. These three swimmers were also were also identified on the basis of physiological responses. Specifically, these individuals were found to have significantly lower levels of muscle glycogen in comparison with the rest of the sample (Costill *et al.* 1988). This depletion was found to be mirrored by a

deficit in daily caloric intake that averaged 1036 kcal. The predictions of overreached or healthy status made on the basis of psychological and physiological information corresponded closely, and the overall agreement between these approaches was 89%. These results support the examination of overtraining and staleness from a multidisciplinary perspective that integrates psychological and physiological assessments. They also underscore the extent of individual differences in the ability of athletes to tolerate intensive physical training.

Mood state responses to training and the staleness syndrome

It has long been known that not all athletes who undergo an intensive training regimen (i.e., overtraining) will benefit from it. In studies of swimmers and other endurance athletes 10–15% have been found to develop the staleness or overtraining syndrome during the course of a season of competitive training (Morgan *et al.* 1987; Raglin & Wilson 1999). Staleness is a condition associated with chronically diminished sport performance that is not rectified by either reductions in training or short-breaks from training. A variety of other signs and symptoms have been reported in stale athletes and among these include medical problems such as infectious disorders, sleep disturbances, changes in appetite, and psychological disturbances, particularly clinical depression (Morgan *et al.* 1987; Kuipers & Keizer 1988; Fry *et al.* 1991; O'Connor 1997). Staleness can be avoided if athletes are prevented from overtraining, but this is not a practical option for serious competitors. Because of this efforts have been made to identify markers that can be reliably used to detect staleness in its early stages, with the goal of using this information to intervene before the disorder becomes fully blown.

The vast majority of monitoring research involved physiological variables and the most commonly studied include heart rate, lactate, ammonia, testosterone, and cortisol (Fry *et al.* 1991). The efficacy of these and other physiological measures has been studied in athletes in the resting state as well as following standardized exercise bouts. Unfortunately, reviews have consistently concluded that evidence for utility of most physiological markers of staleness is uniformly lacking (Kuipers & Keizer 1988; Fry *et al.* 1991; Urhausen 2002). In addition, the responses of these measures may differ in cases of so-called sympathetic or parasympathetic types of staleness (Kuipers & Keizer 1988). Physiological measures are generally expensive, time consuming, and require technical resources beyond those available to most athletes and coaches.

Psychological measures provide a cost-effective and timely alternative, and results of mood state monitoring studies indicate that the POMS can discriminate between stale and healthy athletes. With some exceptions (Morgan *et al.* 1987; Hooper *et al.* 1997) mood disturbances have consistently been found to be higher in athletes showing signs of staleness. These findings appear to generalize to younger athletes as well, and in a report on age group swimmers, Raglin *et al.* (2000) report that swimmers who become stale possessed greater mood disturbance than healthy athletes at all measurement times during the training season.

There is also evidence that the pattern of mood disturbance differs between stale athletes and those who are able to tolerate heavy training loads. Research with college swimmers has revealed that POMS vigor and fatigue factors scores exhibit the largest shift for most athletes, whereas depression is relatively unaffected (Raglin *et al.* 1991). In contrast, depression increases the most of all POMS factors in athletes who develop staleness (see Fig. 6.4).

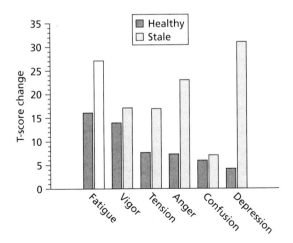

Fig. 6.4 Mean shifts in Profile of Mood State (POMS) variables from easy to hard training in a group of healthy and stale swimmers. Adapted from Raglin *et al.* (1991).

The finding that mood responses can be monitored reliably during overtraining have led researchers to test the feasibility of monitoring mood state in an effort to prevent athletes from becoming stale during a period of intensive training. Morgan *et al.* (reported in Raglin 1993) assessed mood state on a daily basis in collegiate female and male swimmers who were undergoing overtraining. Total mood disturbance scores of each swimmer were contrasted with the team daily and training loads were adjusted for individual swimmers whose scores varied from the team average. In cases in which mood state was at least 1 standard deviation above the team average, the training load was reduced until the total mood disturbance scores declined to a value that differed from the team average by less than 1 standard deviation. Training distance was increased in swimmers who exhibited mood state scores lower than the rest of the team by at least 1 standard deviation. At the end of the season the swimmers were evaluated by the coach and no cases of staleness were reported for the entire sample. While the absence of staleness may simply be a chance occurrence, this was unlikely because in each of the previous 10 seasons the rate of staleness averaged 12% and there were no seasons in which either the men's or women's teams were entirely free from staleness.

As noted earlier, staleness is commonly associated with a host of symptoms, some quite serious. Along with sufficient rest from training, it is important for affected individuals to undergo medical evaluation. Appropriate attention to potential psychological problems is also warranted. Morgan *et al.* (1987) have noted that approximately 80% of stale athletes develop clinical depression of clinical magnitude. These athletes typically require counseling or psychotherapy, sometimes in conjunction with antidepressant medication. Appropriate psychological treatment is important because there is some evidence implicating a biological basis for the depression found in stale athletes (O'Connor *et al.* 1989). Sport psychologists have contended that techniques such as mental imagery or relaxation can be useful in treating staleness (Henschen 1997). Empirical tests of these interventions for staleness have not been conducted, however, and it is recommended that standard medical and psychological treatment be used. Some researchers have proposed that antidepressant medication could be given to athletes as a preventive measure (Armstrong &

VanHeest 2002), but this is not advisable as there is no compelling empirical evidence that such an approach would be effective. Moreover, antidepressant medication is associated with side effects that can compromise the ability of athletes to train intensively, including reduced cardiac output (Martinsen & Stanghelle 1997).

To summarize, endurance athletes possess personality characteristics that are distinct from the general population. Athletes in general have positive mental health profiles and this is particularly true for successful competitors. However, the stress of intense endurance training can alter the mood state of athletes significantly, resulting in mood disturbances in which the psychological profiles of athletes are similar to or even exceed published norms based on nonathlete samples. In the case of athletes who develop the staleness syndrome, the magnitude of mood disturbances is greater and depression of clinical significance is commonly noted (Morgan *et al.* 1987). Some evidence indicates that the use of mood state measures to monitor and adjust training of athletes undergoing intensive training can provide a means of reducing the risk of the staleness syndrome but further research that includes nontreatment control and placebo conditions is needed. Any test of psychological measures with athletes should involve investigators who are trained in their administration and interpretation. It is likely that a monitoring system that incorporates relevant psychological and physiological measures would provide the best chance at identifying stale athletes given the psychobiological nature of the disorder.

Precompetition factors: state anxiety

Research has found that acute psychological states resulting from the stress of impending competition can have a significant impact on sport success. State anxiety responses experienced prior to and during competition have been considered important psychological factors in sport performance. Psychological states are transitory emotions that can change dramatically in intensity from one moment to the next depending on the presence or absence of stressors, the perception and interpretation of these stressors by the individual, and the ability of the individual to cope with stressors.

The traditional perspective held by sport psychologists is that high levels of state anxiety are consistently harmful to performance (Martens *et al.* 1990; LeUnes & Nation 1996; Taylor 1996). As a consequence, the techniques employed in the effort to manipulate anxiety to enhance performance are almost exclusively directed toward reducing anxiety and creating states of relaxation (Taylor 1996). Techniques commonly used toward this end include hypnosis, progressive relaxation, visualization, biofeedback, autogenic training, meditation, negative thought stopping, and confidence enhancement (Martens *et al.* 1990).

The perspective that elevated levels of anxiety are harmful for performance is consistent with several prevailing theories of anxiety and sport performance, the most popular being the inverted-U hypothesis (Martens 1971; Fazey & Hardy 1988; Raglin 1992). According to this explanation, performance is facilitated when anxiety levels are within a moderate range. As anxiety extends above or falls below this range, performance should deteriorate at a progressively greater rate, forming a function in the shape of an inverted-U. The level of skill of an athlete and the nature of the sporting event are believed to influence the optimal moderate range to some degree (Oxendine 1970). As athletes gain in skill it is hypothesized that they should benefit from progressively higher levels of anxiety, but with the inverted-U function being preserved. Conversely, it is assumed that beginners or novice athletes would be most affected by higher anxiety and so the inverted-U function is moved toward the lower end of the anxiety continuum. Sport tasks that are explosive or anaerobic in nature are thought to benefit from a relatively higher level of anxiety compared to endurance sports, whereas tasks requiring minimal physical effort and fine motor control (e.g., archery) should require relatively low levels of anxiety with the inverted-U function between anxiety and performance being preserved in all cases.

Despite the intuitive appeal and long-standing predominance of the inverted-U hypothesis, in recent years it has fallen under considerable criticism. Reviews of both the general psychology literature (Neiss 1988) and sport anxiety research have consistently concluded that the hypothesis is largely invalid, in part because it fails to account for the individual differences in anxiety responses that are frequently observed in sport settings (Raglin 1992; Fazey & Hardy

1992; Hanin 1997). More recent research has provided support for individualized explanations of the influence of anxiety on sport performance. In particular, the Individual Zones of Optimal Functioning (IZOF) model developed by the psychologist Yuri Hanin (1997), based on his research with several thousand athletes, elucidates a relationship between anxiety and sport performance that is totally individualized. The IZOF model proposes that each athlete performs better when her or his level of anxiety falls within an optimal range or zone. Unlike the inverted-U hypothesis and other group-based explanations, according to the IZOF model optimal anxiety can differ considerably across athletes in any given sport, and may range from low to high. In contrast to the inverted-U hypothesis, the IZOF model posits that the skill level of an athlete will not predictably influence the level of anxiety that is optimal for performance. For example, in a group of swimmers with same skill levels competing in the same event, a substantial percentage of individuals should report performing best when anxiety is high, whereas other competitors will benefit from moderate or even low anxiety. IZOF research involving athletes from a variety of endurance supports this prediction. In studies of athletes in swimming and other sports, it has been found that that between 30 and 45% of individuals perform best with high anxiety (Raglin & Hanin 1999), with similar proportions reporting that they benefit from low or moderate anxiety levels. Optimal anxiety values are most commonly determined by having athletes complete an anxiety questionnaire on the basis of how they recalled feeling just prior to their very best performance. Four anxiety units (approximately 0.5 standard deviation) are added and subtracted to this value to yield an optimal anxiety range. Research indicates that there is a moderate to high correlation ($r = 0.60$–0.80) between recalled and actual precompetition anxiety scores, supporting the use of this method for establishing optimal anxiety (Raglin & Hanin 1999).

Before investing time and resources toward helping athletes to regulate their precompetition anxiety, it is crucial to determine the net influence of anxiety and other psychological variables on sport performance. If, for example, research indicates that possessing nonoptimal anxiety levels prior to competition has only a negligible impact on performance, then the time, effort, and potential expense of instituting

anxiety intervention techniques may not be warranted. Some research has been conducted to determine the degree to which performance is influenced by optimal anxiety, as established by IZOF methodology. In a study with adolescent female swimmers, Raglin, Morgan and Wise (1990) examined whether performance differed in cases in which swimmers competed with optimal precompetition anxiety levels that were either optimal or nonoptimal (i.e., above or below the optimal zone). An optimal anxiety zone was established by having each swimmer complete the state portion of the State-Trait Anxiety Inventory (Spielberger *et al.* 1983) on the basis of how she felt "before her very best performance" in accordance with procedures established by Hanin (1986). Actual precompetition anxiety was assessed 1 h before an easy and a difficult dual meet using the same instrument with the standard "right now" instructions. The performance of each swimmer was rated by the coach using a 7-item Likert scale. It was found that athletes rated as performing above average possessed precompetition anxiety levels that were significantly closer to their optimal recalled score compared with swimmers who performed average or below. However, the mean level of precompetition anxiety did not differ between the above and below average performance groups, and this lack of a group trend indicates that the impact of anxiety was individualized and not evident in a group trend toward higher or lower anxiety. In the case of the easy meet, the above and below average performing groups were found to have precompetition anxiety values that diverged from optimal to an equal degree, and it was hypothesized that possessing optimal precompetition anxiety was not crucial for adequate performance in the case of less important competitions. Subsequent work by Salminen *et al.* (1995) also found that optimal precompetition anxiety had a significant impact on performance only in the case of difficult competitions.

In a study that attempted to objectively quantify the net impact of optimal precompetition anxiety on sport performance, Raglin and Turner (1993) found that the performance of track and field athletes was approximately 2.0% ($P < 0.05$) better when anxiety levels fell within the optimal range determined through IZOF procedures. However, when the optimal anxiety was determined on the basis of the inverted-U hypothesis, performance was unchanged. Follow-up research (Turner & Raglin 1996) revealed that the decrement in performance was approximately equal whether anxiety was too low or exceeded optimal values, indicating that the consequences of insufficient anxiety can be as great as when anxiety is excessive. Other more individualized anxiety and performance theories for sport contexts have been recently developed. Primary among these are reversal theory and catastrophe theory. Consistent with the IZOF model, these theories each indicate that anxiety can either facilitate or harm sport performance. However, both reversal and catastrophe theory incorporate specific anxiety or self-reported arousal scales rather than the more general measures used in most IZOF research. Reversal theory (Kerr 1989) contends that self-reported arousal is important to performance, in spite of problems noted in the literature. Arousal is interpreted on the basis of the individual's current hedonic, or emotional state, which in turn is governed by the interaction of "metamotivational states" that exist in opposition. These metamotivational paratelic (high arousal preferring) and telic (low arousal preferring) states can be measured through self-report questionnaires. In summarizing studies that have tested reversal theory in several sports, Kerr and Cox (1991) conclude that more successful athletes report higher levels of arousal than less successful athletes, but experience it as less stressful.

To summarize, anxiety has a significant influence on sport performance. However, its impact is more individualized than what is indicated by traditional approaches, such as the inverted-U hypothesis that predict athletes competing in the same event should exhibit similar responses to anxiety. Research indicates that athletes exhibit considerable variation in the level of anxiety that is most beneficial for their performance. The IZOF model and other recently developed theories of sport anxiety do not support the traditional presumption that high levels of precompetition anxiety are uniformly detrimental to performance. In fact, popular techniques such as relaxation to lower anxiety may result in poorer levels of performance for a significant percentage of athletes, as between 30 and 45% report high anxiety as beneficial for performance. Hence, the indiscriminant use of relaxation or any group-based procedure that results in similar levels of anxiety for an entire team would not benefit all team members and would potentially be counterproductive for a substantial proportion of individuals.

Psychological variables during competition

Research has identified some cognitive factors that have an impact on endurance performance. During competition elite men and women distance runners commonly utilize a cognitive strategy in which attention is directed inward in an attempt to monitor bodily signals. Endurance athletes report paying close attention to sensations such as pain, fatigue, muscle soreness, respiration, and body temperature (Morgan & Pollock 1977). This tactic is described as association; it involves monitoring bodily feedback including kinesthetic sensations and physical exertion, and using this information to regulate pace. There are many anecdotal reports of athletes who have had successful sport performances while associating. In contrast, nonelite athletes adopt a very different cognitive approach during competition (Morgan & Pollock 1977). These individuals use a variety of means to distract themselves from the sensations of physical exertion and discomfort, a strategy referred to as dissociation. Methods used to dissociate may range from simple techniques such as running at the pace of a competitor or repeating a word or phrase in time with pace (e.g., "down"). More unusual examples of dissociation that have been reported include mentally designing and building a house, reliving one's entire education, conducting complex mathematical calculations, and out-of-body experiences where the runner enters the shadow of a competitor (Morgan 1997). There is evidence that dissociation may lengthen the time to exhaustion in steady state endurance tasks, but Morgan (1997) has suggested that the use of dissociation during competition may result in subpar performance.

Some research supports this hypothesis; recreational marathoners who used a dissociative strategy during a race were more likely to "hit the wall" (Stevinson & Biddle 1998). It was speculated that this occurred because the runners were not regulating their pace according to perceived effort and were also underhydrated. In contrast, some researchers have claimed that association is the "riskier" cognitive strategy.

Masters and Ogles (1998) base this contention on their finding that marathoners who routinely associate trained harder, performed better, and had a higher incidence of injury than runners who relied on dissociation. However, the assumption that using association spurs harder and longer training and consequently increases the risk of injury could not be established from the cross-sectional research employed in this study. It seems feasible that more talented athletes simply must associate during competition, just as they must train long and hard if they are to reach their full potential.

Elite athletes do not rely exclusively on association in all situations. Research with elite distance runners has found that approximately 50% reported dissociating exclusively during training, whereas none relied exclusively on dissociation during competition (Morgan et al. 1987, 1988).

Athletes may also differ in the degree to which they monitor bodily feedback accurately during physical exertion. Morgan and Pollock (1997) reported that nonelite runners tended to underrate physical exertion during treadmill running when compared with world-class distance runners. In a study of wrestlers vying for positions on the US Olympic freestyle team, Nagle and colleagues (1975) found that unsuccessful competitors exhibited higher exercise heart rates during standardized exercise testing compared with the wrestlers that were successful in making the team, reflecting fitness differences between the groups. However, perceived exertion ratings did not differ between successful and unsuccessful wrestlers. Morgan (1997) has recently theorized that this finding may indicate that elite athletes are more likely to use association on a routine basis, and not simply during competition. O'Connor (1992) has suggested such differences may arise from the fact that elite athletes associate because they can afford to monitor bodily signals, in part because they are more capable of enduring the discomfort of intense physical effort.

Some research has been conducted to examine the influence of association and dissociation in swimmers (Couture et al. 1999) but this work was marred employing an association technique that had more in common with dissociation. Moreover, the study involved beginning recreational swimmers and its relevance to competitive swimmers is questionable.

Imagery confidence

Various psychological strategies have been advocated to improve sport performance. Among these interventions, mental imagery or visualization is the most widely promoted. Yet despite the popularity of this technique, the benefits associated with imagery appear to be modest at best. A meta-analysis by Feltz and Landers (1983) concluded that "mentally practicing a skill influences performance somewhat better than no practice at all" (p. 25). Reviews of the literature consistently indicate the consequences of imagery are greater for tasks with a significant cognitive component, compared to sporting events in which physical capacity or strength plays a greater role (Feltz & Landers 1983; Driskell et al. 1994).

It is unclear how low-level physiological activity (e.g., electromyography, EMG) would benefit endurance events where performance is limited more by physical conditioning than by fine motor skill or cognitive factors such as memorization. Despite these caveats mental imagery is still advocated for endurance sports, including distance running. In one study cited as evidence for the use of imagery for runners, Burhans (1988) examined the effects of imagery or motivational training to a no-treatment control in adult recreational runners across 12 weeks of training. The rate of improvement in running a 2.4 km (1.5 mile) race was greatest ($P < 0.05$) after 4 weeks of training for the imagery group, but by the end of the training program the improvement was equivalent across conditions. Unfortunately the authors did not include a placebo condition. The special attention inherent in experimental treatments (i.e., the Hawthorne effect) can alter performance significantly (Morgan 1997), and may well account for the short-lived benefits of imagery that were noted in this study. No benefits were associated with the motivational "psyching up" strategy and this finding is consistent with other research involving aerobic endurance activities. Other psychological techniques such as goal setting, arousal management, and cognitive self-regulation have also been promoted for athletes. Reviews of this literature have found that such methods are sometimes associated with performance improvements (Meyers et al. 1996), but important caveats have been acknowledged. Psychological enhancement techniques seldom include appropriate placebo conditions to determine the extent to which changes in performance are simply a consequence of the Hawthorne effect (Morgan 1997). Research on psychological performance enhancement techniques has rarely involved elite athletes (Meyers *et al.* 1996); indeed the majority of studies have comprised "participants with little or no proficiency with the sport task" (p. 157). Also, the endurance activities tested have generally borne little resemblance to actual endurance events.

Conclusions

There is considerable interest in uncovering the factors that contribute to endurance performance. Research to date has largely centered on biological variables. There is evidence that psychological factors also impact endurance performance. Selected personality traits such as emotional stability are associated with success in a variety of sports. Although these findings should not be used in efforts to select athletes for competition, they underscore the impact that mental health has on performance—a fact all too often ignored when considering the needs of the athlete. Other factors such as anxiety also influence sport performance, but at a much more individual level. These findings indicate that psychological research on athletes would benefit from considering the influence of both group and individual factors. Moreover, given the complex nature of endurance performance, a better understanding will come only when psychological and physiological variables are examined conjointly. As stated by the pioneering American sport psychologist Coleman Griffith (1929) some 70 years ago, sport performance involves "the study of vexing physiological and psychological problems, many of which are distorted by the attempt to reduce them to simple terms" (p. vii). Griffith's advice retains its relevance in the case of swimming.

References

APA (1999) *The Standards for Educational and Psychological Testing.* Washington, DC: AERA.

Armstrong, L.E. & VanHeest, J.L. (2002) The unknown mechanism of the overtraining Syndrome clues from depression and psychoneuroimmunology. *Sports Medicine* **32**, 185–209.

Burhans, R.S. (1988) Mental imagery training: effects on running speed performance. *International Journal of Sport Psychology* **19**(1), 26–37.

Cooper, L. (1969) Athletics, activity and personality: a review of the literature. *Research Quarterly* **40**(1), 17–22.

Costill, D.L., Flynn, M.G., Kirwan, J.P., Houmard, J.A., Mitchell, J.B., Thomas, R. & Park, S.H. (1988) Effects of repeated days of intensified training on muscle glycogen and swimming performance. *Medicine and Science in Sports and Exercise* **20**, 249–254.

Couture, R.T., Jerome, W. & Tihanyi, J. (1999) Can associative and dissociative strategies affect the swimming performance of recreational swimmers? *Sport Psychologist* **13**, 334–343.

Driskell, J.E., Copper, C. & Moran, A. (1994) Does mental practice enhance performance? *Journal of Applied Psychology* **79**(4), 481–492.

Dudley, A.T. (1888) The mental qualities of an athlete. *Harvard Alumni Magazine* **6**, 43–51.

Eysenck, H.J., Nias, K.B.D. & Cox, D.N. (1982) Personality and sport. *Advances in Behaviour Research and Therapy* **1**, 1–56.

Fazey, J. & Hardy, L. (1988) *The Inverted-U Hypothesis: A Catastrophe for Sport Psychology?* (BASS Monograph 1). Leeds, UK: White Line Press.

Feltz, D.L. & Landers, D. (1983) Effects of mental practice on motor skill learning and performance: a meta-analysis. *Journal of Sport Psychology* **5**(1), 25–57.

Fry, R.W., Morton, A.R. & Keast, D. (1991) Overtraining in athletes. *Sports Medicine* **12**(1), 32–65.

Griffith, C.R. (1929) *The Psychology of Coaching. Playing the Game.* New York: Charles Scribners' Sons, pp. 83–97.

Hanin, Y.L. (1986) State-trait anxiety research in the USSR. In: C.D. Spielberger & R. Diaz-Guerrero, eds. *Cross Cultural Anxiety, Vol. 3.* Washington, DC: Hemisphere, pp. 45–64.

Hanin, Y.L. (1997) Emotions and athletic performance: individual zones of optimal functioning model. *European Yearbook of Sport Psychology* **1**, 29–72.

Henschen, K.P. (1997) Psychological aspects of over training. In: *Fourth IOC World Congress on Sport Sciences,* Lausanne, Switzerland. International Olympic Committee, p.32.

Hooper, S.L., Traeger Mackinnon, L. & Hanrahan, S. (1997) Mood states as an indication of staleness and recovery. *International Journal of Sport Psychology* **28**(1), 1–12.

Kerr, J.H. (1989) Anxiety, arousal, and sport performance: an application of reversal theory. In: D. Hackfort & C.D. Spielberger, eds. *Anxiety in Sports: An International Perspective.* New York: Hemisphere, pp. 137–151.

Kerr, J.H. & Cox, T. (1991) Arousal and individual differences. *Personality and Individual Differences* **12**, 1075–1085.

Kuipers, H. & Keizer, H.A. (1988) Overtraining in elite athletes: review and directions for the future. *Sports Medicine* **6**, 79–92.

LeUnes, A.D. & Burger, J. (2000) Profile of mood states. Review. *Journal of Applied Sport Psychology* **12**, 5–15.

LeUnes, A.D. & Nation, J.R. (1996) *Sport Psychology: An Introduction*. Chicago: Nelson-Hall.

Mahoney, M.J. (1989) Sport psychology. In: I.S. Cohen, ed. *The G. Stanley Hall Lectures 9*. Washington DC: APA, pp. 101–134.

Martens, R. (1971) Anxiety and motor behavior. *Journal of Motor Behavior* **3**, 151–179.

Martens, R. (1975) Competitive anxiety: theory and research. In: *Proceedings of the 7th Canadian Symposium on Psycho-Motor Learning and Sport Psychology*, Quebec City, pp. 289–292.

Martens, R., Vealey, R.S. & Burton, D. (1990) *Competitive Anxiety in Sport*. Champaign, IL: Human Kinetics.

Martinsen, E.W. & Stanghelle, J.K. (1997) Drug therapy and physical activity. In: W.P. Morgan, ed. *Physical Activity and Mental Health*. Washington, DC: Taylor & Francis, pp. 93–106.

Masters, K.S. & Ogles, B.M. (1998) Associative and dissociative cognitive strategies in exercise and running. *Sport Psychologist* **12**(3), 253–270.

McNair, D.M., Lorr, M. & Droppleman, L.F. (1992) *Profile of Mood States Manual*. San Diego: Educational and Industrial Testing Service.

Meyers, A.W., Whelan, J.P. & Murphy, S.M. (1996) Cognitive behavioral strategies in athletic performance enhancement. In: M. Hersen, R.M. Eisler & P.M. Miller, eds. *Progress in Behavior Modification*. Pacific Grove, CA: Brooks/Cole, pp. 137–164.

Morgan, W.P. (1978a) Sport personology: the credulous-skeptical argument in perspective. In: W.F. Staub, ed. *Sport Psychology: An Analysis of Athlete Behavior*. Ithaca, NY: Movement Publications, pp. 218–227.

Morgan, W.P. (1978b) The credulous-skeptical argument in perspective. In: W.F. Straub, ed. *An Analysis of Athlete Behavior*. Ithaca, NY: Mouvement Publications, pp. 218–227.

Morgan, W.P. (1980a) The trait psychology controversy. *Research Quarterly for Exercise and Sport*, **51**, 50–76.

Morgan, W.P. (1980b) The trait psychology controversy. *Research Quarterly for Exercise and Sport* **51**, 50–76.

Morgan, W.P. (1985) Selected psychological factors limiting performance: a mental health model. In: D.H. Clarke & H.M. Eckert, eds. *Limits of Human Performance*. Champaign, IL: Human Kinetics, pp. 70–80.

Morgan, W.P., Brown, D.L, Raglin, J.S., O'Connor, P.J. & Ellickson, K.A. (1987) Psychological monitoring of overtraining and staleness. *British Journal of Sports Medicine* **21**, 107–114.

Morgan, W.P., O'Connor, P.A., Sparling, P.B. & Pate, R.R. (1987) Psychological characterization of the elite female distance runner. *International Journal of Sports Medicine* **8** (suppl.), 124–131.

Morgan, W.P., O'Connor, P.A., Ellickson, K.A, & Bradley, P.W., (1988) Personality structure, mood states, and performance in elite male distance runners. *International Journal of Sport Psychology* **19**, 247–263.

Morgan, W.P. (1997) Methodological considerations. In: W.P. Morgan, ed. *Physical Activity and Mental Health*. Washington, DC: Taylor & Francis, pp. 3–32.

Morgan, W.P. & Costill, D.L. (1996) Selected psychological characteristics and health behaviors of aging marathon runners: a longitudinal study. *International Journal of Sports Medicine* **17**(4), 305–312.

Morgan, W.P. & Johnson, R.W. (1978) Personality characteristics of successful and unsuccessful oarsmen. *International Journal of Sport Psychology* **9**(2), 119–133.

Morgan, W.P. & Pollock, M.L. (1977) Psychologic characterization of the elite distance runners. In: P. Milvy, ed. *Marathon: Physiological, Medical, Epidemiological, and Psychological Studies, Part 4*. New York: New York Academy of Sciences, pp. 382–403.

Morgan, W.P., Brown, D.R., Raglin, J.S., O'Connor, P.J. & Ellickson, K.A. (1987) Psychological monitoring of overtraining and staleness. *British Journal of Sports Medicine* **21**, 107–114.

Morgan, W.P., Costill, D.L., Flynn, M.G., Raglin, J.S. & O'Connor, P.J. (1988) Mood disturbance following increased training in swimmers. *Medicine and Science in Sports and Exercise* **20**(4), 408–414.

Nagle, F.J., Morgan, W.P., Hellickson, R.O., Serfas, R.C. & Alexander, J.F. (1975) Spotting success traits in Olympic contenders. *Physician and Sports Medicine* **3**(12), 31–34.

Newcombe, P.A. & Boyle, G.J. (1995) High school students' sports personalities: Variations across participation level, gender, type of sport, and success. *International Journal of Sport Psychology* **26**(3), 277–294.

Neiss, R. (1988) Reconceptualizing arousal: psychobiological states in motor performance. *Psychological Bulletin* **103**, 345–366.

O'Connor, P.J. (1992) Psychological aspects of endurance performance. In: R.J. Shephard & P.O. Astrand, eds. *Endurance in Sport*. Oxford: Blackwell Scientific, pp. 139–145.

O'Connor, P.J. (1997) Overtraining and staleness. In: W.P. Morgan, ed. *Physical Activity and Mental Health*. Washington, DC: Taylor & Francis, pp. 149–160.

O'Connor, P.J., Morgan, W.P. & Raglin, J.S. (1991) Psychobiological effects of 3 days of increased training in female and male swimmers. *Medicine and Science in Sports and Exercise* **23**, 1055–1061.

O'Connor, P.J., Morgan, W.P., Raglin, J.S., Barksdale, C.M. & Kalin, N.H. (1989) Mood state and salivary cortisol changes following overtraining in female swimmers. *Psychoneuroendocrinology* **14**, 303–310.

Ostrow, A.C. (1990) *Directory of Psychological Tests in the Sport and Exercise Sciences*. Morgantown, WV: Fitness Information Technology, Inc.

Oxendine, J.B. (1970) Emotional arousal and motor performance. *Quest* **13**, 23–32.

Raglin, J.S. (1992) Anxiety and sport performance. In: J.O. Holloszy, ed. *Exercise and Sport Sciences Reviews* 20. New York: Williams & Wilkins, pp. 243–274.

Raglin, J.S. (1993) Overtraining and staleness: Psychometric monitoring of endurance athletes. In: R.B. Singer, M. Murphey & L.K. Tennant, eds. *Handbook of Research on Sport Psychology*. New York: Macmillan, pp. 840–850.

Raglin, J.S. (2001) Psychological factors in sport performance: the mental health model revisited. *Sports Medicine* **31**, 875–890.

Raglin, J.S. & Hanin, Y.L. (1999) Competitive anxiety. In: Y.L. Hanin, ed. *Emotions in Sport*. Champaign, IL: Human Kinetics, pp. 93–111.

Raglin, J.S. & Morgan, W.P. (1994) Development of a scale for use in monitoring training-induced distress in athletes. *International Journal of Sports Medicine* **15**, 84–88.

Raglin, J.S. & Turner, P.E. (1993) Anxiety and performance in track and field athletes: a comparison of the inverted-U hypothesis with zone of optimal functioning theory. *Personality and Individual Differences* **14**, 163–171.

Raglin, J.S. & Wilson, G.S. (1999) Overtraining in athletes. In: Y.L.Hanin, ed. *Emotion in Sports*. Champaign, IL: Human Kinetics, pp. 191–207.

Raglin, J.S., Morgan, W.P. & O'Connor, P.J. (1991) Changes in mood states during training in female and male college swimmers. *International Journal of Sports Medicine* **12**, 585–589.

Raglin, J.S., Morgan, W.P. & Wise, K. (1990) Pre-competition anxiety in high school girls swimmers: a test of optimal function theory. *International Journal of Sports Medicine* **11**, 171–175.

Raglin, J.S., Sawamura, S., Alexiou, S., Hassmen, P. & Kentta, G. (2000) Training practices and staleness in 13–18-year-old swimmers: a cross-cultural study. *Pediatric Exercise Science* **12**(1), 61–70.

Rushall, B.S. (1970) An investigation of the relationship between personality variables and performance categories in swimmers. *International Journal of Sport Psychology* **1**(2), 93–104.

Salminen, S., Liukkonen, J., Hanin, Y. & Hyvonen, A. (1995) Anxiety and athletic performance of Finnish athletes: an application of zone of optimal functioning model. *Personality and Individual Differences* **19**, 725–729.

Smith, T.W. (1997) Punt, pass, and ponder the questions. *The New York Times*, April 20, F-11.

Spielberger, C.D., Gorsuch, R.L., Lushene, R.E., Vagg, P.R. & Jacobs, G.A. (1983) *Manual for the State-Trait Anxiety Inventory STAI (Form Y)*. Palo Alto, CA: Consulting Psychologists Press.

Stevinson, C.D. & Biddle, S.J. (1998) Cognitive orientations in marathon running and "hitting the wall." *British Journal of Sports Medicine* **32**(3), 229–234.

Taylor, J. (1996) Intensity regulation and athletic performance. In: J.L. Van Raalte & B.W. Brewer, eds. *Exploring Sport and Exercise Psychology*. Washington, DC: APA, pp. 75–106.

Turner, P.E. & Raglin, J.S. (1996) Variability in precompetition anxiety and performance in college track and field athletes. *Medicine and Science in Sports and Exercise* **28**(3), 378–385.

Urhausen, A. (2002) Diagnosis of overtraining: what tools do we have? *Sports Medicine* **32**(2), 95–102.

Urhausen, A., Gabriel, H. & Kindermann, W. (1995) Blood hormones as markers of training stress and overtraining. *Sports Medicine* **20**(4), 251–276.

Vanden Auweele, Y., Cuyper, D.D., Mele, V.V. & Tzewnicki, R. (1993) Elite performance and personality: from description and prediction to diagnosis and intervention. In: R.N. Singer, M. Murphey & L.K. Tennant, eds. *Handbook of Research on Sport Psychology*. New York: Macmillan, pp. 257–289.

Verde, T., Thomas, S. & Shepard, R. (1992) Potential markers of heavy training in highly trained distance runners. *British Journal of Sports Medicine* **26**, 167–175.

Warburton, F.W. & Kane, J.E. (1966) Personality related to sport and physical ability. In: J.E. Kane, ed. *Readings in Physical Education*. London: Physical Education Association of Great Britain and Northern Ireland, pp. 61–89.

Chapter 7
Medical issues related to swimming

David F. Gerrard

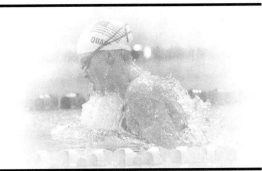

Asthma

Asthma describes a very common clinical condition recognized in many young aquatic athletes who have reached the highest international levels. For athletes, their parents, and coaches, asthma should not equate to a life of restricted physical capacity. Contemporary treatment regimes achieve high levels of control, and the cornerstone to effective asthma management is education. It is exceedingly important for coaches and swimmers to be very familiar with the cause of asthma, its management and, of course, avoidance of any potential "triggers." Indoor swimming pools present additional challenges as a result of the chemicals used for disinfection and their subsequent reaction with ammonia from body fluids such as urine and sweat. Chlorination produces compounds like chloramines and many other potential irritants that may provoke respiratory, eye, and skin problems in sensitive swimmers.

What is asthma?

In simple terms, asthma infers an increased sensitivity of the lining of the airways—a sensitive combination of hair-lined epithelium, mucus-secreting cells, and smooth muscle. "Hyperresponsive" or "twitchy" airways (bronchi) when stimulated produce increased amounts of mucus, become locally inflamed, and are caused to constrict as the result of smooth muscle action. This latter phenomenon is referred to as "bronchospasm." To the asthmatic swimmer these changes combine to reduce the cross-sectional area of the bronchi resulting in restricted lung function and an audible "wheeze" on forced expiration.

Asthma sufferers are highly sensitive to such things as dust, pollens, animal fur, cigarette smoke, or cold air. Frequently there is an accompanying family history of eczema (dermatitis), hay fever, or seasonal allergy. In some cases *exercise-induced asthma* is the working diagnosis, reflective of the link with physical activity. Of all activities though, swimming is widely recognized as being least provocative—one reason for swimming to attract such a large number of asthma sufferers. Contrary to popular misconception it is possible for a well-controlled asthmatic swimmer to excel; in fact there are examples of asthmatics winning Olympic and World swimming titles.

The diagnosis of asthma

Asthma is suspected in anyone for whom breathing becomes restricted or provoked by any one of the triggering factors mentioned earlier. On the basis of such a history a routine medical examination is mandatory and tests of lung function are necessary to confirm an accurate clinical diagnosis. These involve tests of airway responsiveness to the specific challenges of hypertonic saline, methacholine, and exercise. Evidence of the reversibility of bronchospasm in response to specific inhaled drugs requires interpretation by a specialist respiratory physician before a definite diagnosis can be made. Any competitive athlete diagnosed with asthma must retain a copy of his or her respiratory function tests for future declaration at the time of doping control to justify the use of antiasthma medication that is on the International Olympic Committee (IOC) and the World Anti-Doping Agency (WADA) list of restricted drugs.

Antiasthma drugs

In a general sense, medication to treat asthma is designed to achieve immediate control ("reliever" drugs) or long-term control ("preventer" drugs). Physicians base asthma drug management on combinations of these two types of medication. Relievers are those that relax smooth muscle and help reduce mucus production while the preventers are essentially anti-inflammatory agents.

The current IOC and WADA list permits the use of the following drugs where the diagnosis of asthma has been confirmed:

1 *Beta-2 agonists* (by inhalation only): these are reliever drugs
- Salbutamol
- Terbutaline
- Salmeterol
- Formoterol

2 *Glucocorticosteroids* (by inhalation only): these are preventer drugs
- Beclomethasone
- Budesonide
- Dexamethasone
- Flunisolide
- Triamcinolone

It always remains the responsibility of any athlete to check their medication to ensure that what they have been prescribed is on the permitted list. Your national sports drug agency has updated information readily available.

Anemia

By definition, anemia describes a reduced number of red blood cells (RBCs) or a reduction in hemoglobin (Hb) concentration. A number of factors may be responsible and the consequence of chronic, untreated anemia is inappropriate fatigue, which for the aquatic athlete frequently translates into an inexplicable loss of form. The Hb component of the RBC has a strong affinity for oxygen. Tightly bound to Hb and

transported via blood, oxygen is thereby made available to working muscles. There are several categories of anemia, classified according to the size of the RBC. But for the sake of this discussion we will concentrate on the anemia commonly seen in athletes.

Causes of anemia

Iron is the essential building block of hemoglobin and this important element should come from daily food sources. Iron deficiency causes the commonest form of anemia, in athletes. Microscopically, the RBCs appear small (microcytic) and pale (hypochromic). Dietary iron must first be absorbed and then incorporated into the RBCs (erythrocytes)—part of the process of RBC manufacture termed erythropoiesis and stimulated by the hormone erythropoietin (EPO) and occurring chiefly in the marrow of long bones and the kidney. Quite simply there are three factors responsible for this type of anemia: the first is insufficient dietary iron, the second is poor iron absorption, and third, iron loss, most frequently by excessive blood loss.

Diagnosis of anemia

A clinical diagnosis is made on the basis of suspicion (a history of relevant symptoms) confirmed by physical examination (revealing typical signs) and appropriate investigations (in this case blood tests). In the case of anemia this is a little more difficult because swimmers in heavy training although naturally fatigued are not necessarily all anemic. Medical opinion and laboratory investigations are essential to confirm the diagnosis. The following case history offers a typical picture of the anemic athlete.

CASE STUDY

Amy, a 17-year-old competitive swimmer became inexplicably tired and began to lose interest in her sport and studies because of extreme tiredness and poor performance. Her moods altered and she began to shun friends and teammates. At the request of her parents and coach she accepted medical advice. An astute sports physician asked Amy about her diet and menstrual pattern. She confessed to becoming "vegetarian" a year earlier and described menstrual cycles that had become erratic, much heavier, and very painful over the previous 6 months. Amy had lost weight (4 kg), looked very pale, and was provisionally diagnosed as being anemic due to iron deficiency. Subsequent blood tests revealed a low Hb level with supportive evidence of depleted serum iron and iron stores (ferritin).

Amy was commenced on a course of oral iron tablets, given sound nutritional advice (sources of iron in a vegetarian menu), and commenced on a low dose, oral contraceptive pill to control her heavy periods. Within 3 months she responded to the iron supplementation, her periods became regular and lighter, and she had incorporated one red meat meal into her weekly diet. She returned to full swim training and follow-up blood results showed a significant improvement in Hb levels and iron stores. Within one season she had regained previous competitive form.

Treatment of anemia

The mainstay of treating iron deficiency is clearly to correct the imbalance of iron intake against losses. This usually involves oral iron supplementation with concurrent administration of vitamin C to enhance iron absorption. At the same time it is essential that attention be paid to the diet of the athlete. Sources of iron in the diet are either "heme" (red meats, poultry, fish) or "nonheme" (whole grain cereals, vegetables). The former group is recommended but those with strong vegetarian beliefs can still achieve significant iron gains. Foods high in tannin (tea) or phytate (fiber) should be avoided since these block the uptake of iron. And finally where there is a demonstrable cause of excessive blood loss (such as heavy periods) it is appropriate to control this mechanism of iron depletion.

It is important to stress that the inappropriate use of iron supplements on scant symptomatic evidence should be strongly discouraged. Excessive iron can have very serious consequences for individuals with the inherited disorder of hemochromatosis. About 5–8 individuals in 1000 have this genetic trait, with a male–female ratio of 5:1. Indiscriminate iron supplementation in these individuals may cause iron-containing pigment to deposit in the liver, heart, joints, and the skin.

KEY POINTS

- Iron deficiency is the commonest cause of anemia in swimmers
- The accurate diagnosis demands special blood tests
- Treatment involves iron supplements and nutritional advice
- Sensible vegetarian diets still provide sufficient iron
- Red meats, fish, and poultry are the richest sources of "hem" iron
- Unsubstantiated use of iron supplements may be dangerous

The ears, eyes, nose, and throat in swimmers

Exposure to water, frequently chlorinated and often contaminated by human perspiration, urine, body lotion, and hair spray, may predispose swimmers to problems of their upper respiratory tracts, ears, and eyes. There are a number of conditions that swimmers and their coaches should be wary of. For the most part these are preventable or at least eminently treatable if the early symptoms are recognized.

Swimmer's ear (otitis externa)

Many microorganisms thrive in a warm, moist environment. The swimmer's ear canal provides such a setting—ideal for the growth of bacteria with exotic names like *Pseudomonas aeruginosa*, *Staphylococcus aureus*, or *Escherichia coli*. However, the name of the organism is far less important than recognizing the symptoms and acknowledging the need for treatment. Swimmers will experience pain and itching of the outer ear that frequently invites relief from inserting such things as cotton buds into the ear. This practice irritates the lining of the canal (causing local damage) and impacts naturally produced earwax, deep in the canal (Fig. 7.1). Trapped moisture stimulates bacterial growth with subsequent infection. Tenderness of the outer shell of the ear with evidence of localized skin infection is also a common accompaniment.

Treatment requires a combination of antibiotic and anti-inflammatory (corticosteroid) application either in drop or ointment form. After swimming, the use of drops of a drying agent is also helpful. A mixture of equal parts of isopropyl alcohol and acetic acid is frequently prescribed. The additional use of soft earplugs and well-fitting caps will also protect the ear canal from moisture. In severe chronic cases it may be necessary to keep the swimmer out of the water for up to 2 weeks. Using a hair dryer to keep the outer canal and shells of the ear dry is another helpful tip.

Otitis media

Otitis media is an infection of the middle ear chamber. Swimmers may complain of earache, dizziness, and a hearing loss. There may be evidence of an associated

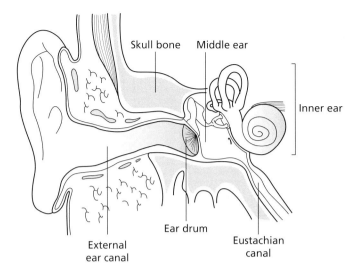

Fig. 7.1 Anatomy of the ear: cross section.

upper respiratory tract (URT) infection resulting in blockage of the eustachian tubes that connect the middle ear to the back of the throat. Uncontrolled pressure within the middle chamber causes the eardrum to bulge, with the imminent risk of rupture. Treatment involves antibiotic use together with decongestants that are available in many forms. For chronic sufferers of otitis media it may become necessary for a specialist to insert small tubes (grommets) in the eardrum to assist drainage. Swimming may continue even when grommets have been inserted but the use of a combined preparation of antibiotic and anti-inflammatory eardrops will help decrease the incidence of infection. Swimmers must confine themselves to surface swimming and be cautioned against diving underwater (such as in synchronized swimming or diving) where increased pressure could cause the spread of infection.

Swimmer's exostoses (osteomata)

After many years of being immersed in water—especially cool water—many swimmers' ears develop what are termed "exostoses." These are small outcrops of very hard bone that grow from the inner walls of the external ear canal. The bone growth, stimulated by the cool water, may obstruct the canal so that water becomes trapped. The skin becomes irritated and local infection may develop. In some cases the canal

becomes completely occluded, hearing is impaired, and a delicate, complicated surgical procedure is necessary to clear the offending bony obstruction. Unfortunately little can be done to prevent the development of these exostoses apart from wearing caps and avoiding cold water. Many surfers, particularly those from the more temperate parts of the world are frequently affected by this condition. The use of soft malleable ear plugs is strongly recommended.

Conjunctivitis

Inflammation of the sensitive membrane that covers the scelra (white) of the eye and the inside of the eyelids is called conjunctivitis (Fig. 7.2). In swimmers it usually causes an irritating "gritty" sensation with an annoying discharge. It is the result of local insult either from direct trauma, infection, or allergy. The signs deserve assessment by an experienced physician. A thick creamy discharge would typically indicate bacterial infection while a watery discharge usually indicates an allergic reaction. The potential for viral infection (such as herpes simplex) must never be overlooked and carries a high risk of spread to other swimmers.

Treatment options are based entirely on the diagnosis. Topical antibiotics are used for bacterial infection, corticosteroids or antihistamines for allergies, and antiviral agents for herpes infection. Swim goggles

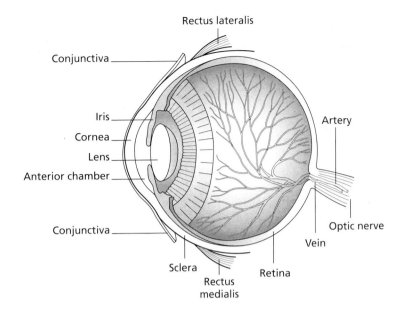

Rectus lateralis

Conjunctiva

Iris

Cornea

Lens

Anterior chamber

Conjunctiva

Artery

Optic nerve

Vein

Sclera

Rectus
medialis

Retina

Fig. 7.2 Anatomy of the eye: cross
section.

have reduced the frequency of eye problems, but
localize impact injuries have resulted from goggles
on elastic straps being flicked back against the eye
socket.

Pterygia

A pterygium is a clear growth of thin tissue that grows
on the eye from the nasal corner across to meet the
pupil. These benign growths are frequently seen in
open water swimmers and surfers, whose eyes have
been continuously irritated by ultraviolet light (sun)
and wind and tiny particles of dust or sand. Frequently,
pterygia become richly supplied by small blood vessels
that give the eye a "blood-shot" appearance. On reaching the nasal margin of the pupil a pterygium might
continue to grow and ultimately affect vision. They
do not regress naturally and require surgical removal.
However if the stimuli continue, pterygia may recur.
The use of appropriate UVL-protective sunglasses is
strongly advised.

Sinusitis

The URT includes the nose, mouth, the sinuses, and
throat, extending down to the start of the trachea. This
sensitive tract is lined by a delicate mucous membrane

that is prone to infection from bacterial and viral
causes. The sinuses are special air sacs situated behind the nose and extending up behind the eyes. They
warm and humidify the air we breathe and trap small
foreign particles like dust and pollen. If the sinus lining
becomes inflamed, the small drainage portals (ostia)
become blocked and the sinuses become filled with
mucous infected by aerobic bacteria such as *Strepo-
tococcus* and *Haemophilus* species. Swimmers are frequently prone to acute sinusitis. The symptoms may
include a feeling of URT congestion, fullness behind
the eyes, and headaches. Chronic sinusitis leaves the
sufferer feeling very miserable, often with a thick nasal
discharge, and a productive cough at night or when lying face up (supine).

Treatment demands an accurate diagnosis and advice from an ENT specialist. The aims are to open the
ostia, clear the trapped mucus, and treat the underlying disorder. Medications that decongest the swollen
mucosa may facilitate drainage and antibiotics used
judiciously ought to kill the bacteria. There are many
acceptable decongestants that contain no banned substances. If this treatment is unsuccessful, special sinus X-rays or a CT scan may be necessary to delineate
the area of sinus infection. In chronic cases, referral
to a specialist is necessary and in some cases surgical
drainage may be necessary.

Injury prevention in young aquatic athletes

Aquatic athletes usually begin training at an early age, before their musculoskeletal systems have matured. There is the potential for injury if a young swimmer's progress is too rapid or unmonitored. Overuse is the common injury mechanism for the young swimmer who is particularly prone to problems of the shoulder (rotator cuff muscles), the low back, and the knee joint. Sports physicians now recognize swimming-specific conditions such as *swimmer's shoulder, butterfly swimmer's back,* and *breaststroker's knee*. Coaches not only play an integral part in recognizing the early indicators of these injuries but they can help to prevent them by monitoring training load, and also by paying particular attention to stroke mechanics, weight training, or other dryland programs. Although this section deals specifically with injuries in swimmers, the discussion applies equally to water polo players, synchronized swimmers, and in many cases divers.

The young skeleton

Because so many injuries have their genesis in younger swimmers, it is helpful to have an understanding of the immature musculoskeletal system. The skeleton represents a bony scaffold for the attachment of soft tissues (muscles, tendons, and ligaments). During preadolescence the skeleton undergoes rapid growth, a fact of particular significance to injury. Sport-related injuries are universally classified according to their mechanism. There are those caused by acute trauma and those that result from minor, repetitive stress, or "overuse." The latter represent the injuries most commonly seen in swimming. Their early recognition and active management will minimize the potential for chronic disability and interrupted training.

Growth site injury

At the ends of the long bones are regions called the *epiphyses* or growth plates. These are sites of new bone formation, from which bone length increases. Where two bones come together, the resulting articulation is called a joint and there are unique characteristics associated with the joints of young athletes. *Synovial joints*, such as the shoulder, knee, and elbow, possess a specialized covering of articular cartilage over adjacent bone ends that are primed to accommodate rapid growth. Like the epiphyses, this cartilage is prone to damage from repetitive overuse. Any young swimmer who complains of pain in the region of a joint or growth plate deserves medical investigation. Another site of potential injury in the young swimmer is at the attachment of tendon to bone. These sites are called *apophyses,* and are very vulnerable to the constant pull or traction of tendons during the repetition of swim training. A common apophyseal site of overuse is at the front of the knee where the tendon of the quadriceps (thigh) muscles attaches to the upper tibia (shin).

Overuse injuries

Given their level of activity, all swimmers are at risk of overuse or repetitive stress injury. Young musculoskeletal systems normally heal very quickly and with an accurate, early diagnosis, the disruption to training is usually minimal. Swimmers may present with overuse injuries such as tendinitis (inflamed tendons) at sites around the knee joint or shoulder where tendon or muscle attachments are exposed to repetitive traction or pulling forces. Recovery depends upon the severity of the original injury, correct management, and the swimmer's willingness to follow a realistic rehabilitation program.

Specific sites of swimming injury

The shoulder

Anatomy of the shoulder

Of all the joints in the body, the shoulder is the most mobile (Fig. 7.3). It is capable of an extraordinary range of movement because of the relationship of the head of the humerus and the shallow cup (glenoid fossa) of the scapula that is deepened by a rim of fibrous connective tissue. A firm capsule, reinforced by thickenings (ligaments) that stabilize the joint completes this "ball-and-socket" relationship. It offers a unique range of movement in all planes. Understanding the relationship of the bones, muscles, tendons, and ligaments around the shoulder will help the swimmer and coach respect the potential for injury and recognize the structures most likely to be implicated.

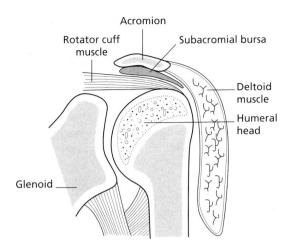

Acromion

Rotator cuff
muscle

Subacromial bursa

Deltoid
muscle

Humeral
head

Glenoid

Fig. 7.3 Anatomy of the shoulder joint: cross section.

The head of the humerus and the glenoid fossa of the scapula (shoulder blade) constitute the anatomical shoulder joint, but overhanging this is the acromion process and its articulation with the clavicle (collarbone). Immediately below is a soft, fluid-filled cushion named the subacromial bursa. Next is the attachment of a group of muscles called the *rotator cuff*. These muscles are important in holding the humerus in its socket and carry a large amount of the stress associated with the shoulder action of freestyle and butterfly.

Swimmer's shoulder

Pain in the shoulder of the competitive swimmer is common. It may begin with an irritating "niggle" associated with training or progress to pain that lingers on after exercise, to become persistent, even at rest. This latter stage reflects chronic irritation of one or more of the soft tissue structures around the shoulder. It is the result of repetitive arm strokes—calculated by some authorities as about 2 million per year in a serious competitive swimmer. The tendons of the rotator cuff, especially the *supraspinatus*, are commonly implicated in this condition, but the long biceps tendon is also frequently involved. The resultant inflammatory process may cause thickening of the tendons as they pass beneath the *acromion process* causing what is referred to as an "impingement syndrome" of the subacromial space.

When examining the painful shoulder of a swimmer, the physician takes into account several possible contributions to the problem, including stroke mechanics and even the choice of breathing side. Unusual prominence of the bony acromion process, imbalance between the major muscle groups around the shoulder, and abnormal movement (instability) of the shoulder are common findings. Examination by plain X-rays, ultrasound, CT scan, or MRI will enable the physician to confirm or exclude likely causes of shoulder pain.

When a diagnosis has been established, a number of treatment options are available. The first is to avoid the specific mechanics of the offending stroke and to correct obvious muscle imbalance around the shoulder. This does not necessarily mean complete rest, but rather it involves selective activities to minimize the potential for "detraining." Swimmers may maintain water work through kicking drills, nonaggravating strokes, and limited dryland workouts. The assessment of swimming technique involves the use of video analysis and biomechanical interpretation that should identify any imbalance. The use of hand paddles has also been recognized as provoking shoulder pain, as has the posture associated with the use of kickboards. Treatment by physical measures such as "ice massage" to the shoulder immediately after training is often helpful. Other physical therapy modalities including ultrasound may also provide temporary relief. Medication to reduce the pain and inflammation is also frequently prescribed in the form of oral, nonsteroidal anti-inflammatory agents (NSAIAs). Particular benefit is reported from the use of the new generation of "COX 2 specific" NSAIAs. However, these medications should only be taken in accordance with strict medical supervision.

Obviously where conservative measures fail invasive alternatives may become necessary. In some cases, localized injections of corticosteroid (hydrocortisone) are indicated. Infrequently, surgery is necessary and includes the use of decompressive techniques to relieve pressure in the subacromial space, simple debridement of rotator cuff tears (more common in master swimmers), or stabilization of the shoulder where gross hypermobility or frank instability has been identified.

But clearly, by far the best method to overcome the problem of swimmer's shoulder is to recognize the early signs, make necessary technical changes, take rest, consult with medical support staff and prevent the symptoms from progressing to the stage of chronic pain, and disruption of training. This condition is also reported in the shoulders of water polo players.

The knee

The knee joint is the next most common site of injury in swimmers. In water polo and synchronized swimming the provocative "egg-beater" kick is a frequent cause of knee pain in much the same way that the "whip kick" of breaststroke may also provoke discomfort.

Unlike the shoulder, the knee joint is a "hinge" with a much more restricted range of movement limited to one plane. The flattened upper end (*plateau*) of the tibia with two discs of cartilage (*menisci*) articulates with the rounded condyles of the lower femur. Four strong ligaments provide stability to this rather incongruous joint. These are the collateral ligaments—the medial on the inner side of the knee, the lateral on the outer side, and two internal ligaments that cross the joint internally. The latter are the cruciate ligaments—far more frequently injured in the deceleration trauma of weight-bearing sports. Overlaying this arrangement are the strong quadriceps muscles on the front of the thigh and the hamstrings, their posterior-placed counterparts. External to the knee joint but important to the function of the quadriceps mechanism is the patella (kneecap), which glides in the *intercondylar notch* of the femur and is attached above to the quadriceps tendon and below via the patellar tendon into the front of the tibia.

Breaststroker's knee

The specific "whip-kick" action of breaststroke is widely recognized as the most likely cause of this problem. The "knock-kneed" or *valgus* stress demanded by this kick compares to the stress of the "egg-beater" action of the kick frequently employed by water polo players and synchronized swimmers. Repetitive stretching of the medial collateral ligament causes localized pain over the inner side of the knee. In some cases this may be complicated by damage to the medial meniscus, a diagnosis considered where the pain is more localized to the medial joint margin or where there may be mechanical "locking" of the joint. A third possible cause of medial knee pain is the common attachment of three muscles to an area of the upper medial tibia called the *pes anserinus* associated with a

small bursa that may also become inflamed and give rise to very local pain aggravated by any valgus stress, such as the breaststroke kick. It becomes self evident to the sufferer of these conditions that continuing aggravation is not an option. Rest from the offending kicking action is essential but the swimmer may maintain cardiorespiratory fitness using other strokes or "arms only" and "pull-buoy" drills. Ice massage and physical therapy modalities are often successful in moderating acute knee pain and NSAIAs are also indicated with the usual caution. Apart from the need to excise an offending portion of torn meniscus, the need for surgery in these cases is not commonly indicated.

Anterior knee pain

Abnormal "tracking" of the patella in its groove on the femur causes another relatively common source of pain over the front (anterior) of the knee. This condition is referred to as the "patello-femoral compartment syndrome" caused by repetitious movements of the kneecap in the flexion/extension kicking pattern of all four strokes, but particularly breaststroke. Swimmers frequently describe pain when they sit for long periods (also known as "movie-goer's knee") or when they walk up and down stairs. A feeling of "grating" beneath the kneecap is a common accompaniment but bears little reflection on the severity of the problem. In many, the kneecap is very mobile and the inner belly of the quadriceps (vastus medialis) is poorly developed. This creates a pattern of poor "patellar tracking" and is a well-recognized diagnostic sign more common in female swimmers.

Treatment of the unstable patella may begin with specific exercises to correct the pull of the quadriceps muscles. External forms of bracing have their place but provide little more than temporary relief if the main cause is not addressed. Patellar stabilizing braces or locally applied taping techniques help to realign the patella but these are interim measures. Symptomatic relief may also be obtained from the use of ice massage, physical therapy, or NSAIAs. In rare cases, surgery is indicated for those with grossly unstable kneecaps that become prone to spontaneous dislocation.

The lower back

Many sports place recurrent, stressful demands on the low back from repetitive actions that frequently involve hyperextension and rotation. The structures

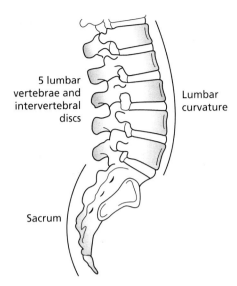

Fig. 7.4 Anatomy of the spine—lower back: cross section.

most likely to be affected are muscles and their sheaths (myofascial tissue), the immature portions of the vertebral bodies, or the spongy intervertebral discs (Fig. 7.4). In some sports there is also a well-described pattern of bony stress that can lead to the production of fine hairline breaks referred to as "stress" or "fatigue" fractures.

In strokes that involve repetitive hyperextension (back arching) or in some of the more explosive synchronized swimming routines, the risk of low back problems must always be considered. Where there is the added element of rapid rotation the risk of damage increases. As routines become more demanding the need for expert coaching is important, particularly in the young swimmer whose bones and muscles are still immature.

Butterfly swimmer's back

The butterfly stroke demands repetitive lumbo-sacral hyperextension to facilitate the traditional "dolphin" kick. This action, repeated many times in training is accentuated during the breathing phase. As a consequence many young butterfly swimmers are troubled by chronic low backache that may be caused by stress on a variety of structures. These include muscles, lumbo-sacral and sacroiliac ligaments, the small "facet" joints between vertebrae, the developing vertebrae themselves, or the intervertebral discs. Chronic low back pain in an adolescent athlete should always

be fully investigated. Specialized radiological techniques such as CT scanning or magnetic resonance imaging MRI will rule out bony injury and also demonstrate the integrity of the surrounding soft tissues, including the intervertebral discs. Plain X-rays of the lower spine to include specific lateral oblique views are still considered to be the most economic means to demonstrate localized bone stress in lumbar vertebrae. The overloaded regions of bone "fatigue" are described as sites of *spondylolysis*—an overuse injury in young tennis players, volleyball strikers, and cricket fast bowlers. They are not common in young butterfly swimmers but should always be ruled out when unremitting low back pain is made worse by hyperextension and rotation of the lumbar spine. Occasionally, bilateral stress fractures of the *pars interarticularis* may cause one vertebra to slip forward on its neighbor, resulting in a condition known as a *spondylolisthesis*. This condition may have serious long-term consequences and should always be reviewed by an orthopedic specialist. Other common causes of low back pain in butterfly swimmers include muscle or ligamentous strain. These are diagnosed by careful examination associated with typical clinical features. The thoracic spine of the adolescent may also be the site of a condition called "Scheuermann's disease"—a developmental condition treated symptomatically and not linked to any sinister, long-term implications. Rehabilitation of the swimmer's back demands a multidisciplinary approach with contributions from coach, physical therapist, and physician. Posture, hamstring tightness, trunk mobility, and lumbar spine stability must be assessed. Strengthening and stabilization techniques are helpful. Where injury to bone is suspected, close medical scrutiny is recommended.

The synchronized swimmer's lower back

Some of the more explosive routines that have become a feature of contemporary synchronized swimming competition include elements that place great stress on the lumbar intervertebral discs. Where there is an existing "weakness" of a particular disc, a rupture of the ring of fibrous tissue containing the soft disc contents may occur as a disc "prolapse" or bulge. This has the potential to irritate sensitive structures including nearby nerve roots. Aggravation results in acute pain often referred along the course of the particular nerve root. The condition of "sciatica" is reflective of pain that radiates down the buttock but having its origin in the low back where nerve roots are irritated. Medical management of all back problems may include various physical or manual modalities and in some instances appropriate prescribed medication to relieve pain, muscle spasm, and inflammation. The cornerstone of effective treatment is an accurate diagnosis.

Other medical conditions (nonorthopedic)

Infectious mononucleosis (glandular fever)

Infectious mononucleosis (IM) is a chronic viral infection widely reported in preadolescence where droplet, respiratory spread of the Epstein–Barr (EB) virus is enhanced by close contact. Groups of adolescents and young adults brought together in University halls of residence, military establishments, or in sports teams are commonly affected. Typical early signs include a flu-like illness with a sore throat, fever, muscle or joint aches, and inappropriate tiredness. For the competitive swimmer there may be an inexplicable "loss of form," frequently attributed (by significant others) to a psychological cause. Meanwhile the swimmer experiences increasing tiredness that, despite extra rest, may progress to a loss of appetite and a frequent lack of motivation for training, academic, and social activities. Uncharacteristic mood changes often signal the need for medical intervention. On examination, a physician will commonly find enlarged lymph glands at various sites and there may be clinical evidence of a painfully enlarged liver.

The clinical suspicion of IM is confirmed by specific blood tests that indicate the body's recognition of a viral infection and a subsequent immune response. This pattern of infection is accompanied by an increase in the population of white blood cells called monocytes, from which this condition derives its name. IM is a "rate-limiting" rather than a serious "life-threatening" infection. In very simple terms, exposure to the EB virus stimulates an immune response as a natural defense mechanism. Liver and spleen enlargement reflect antibody production and virus destruction, while swollen, tender, lymph glands demonstrate the body's *immune competence*—the ability to

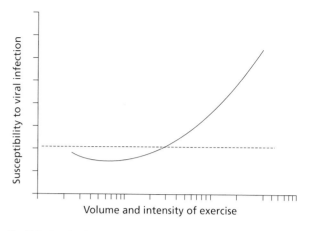

Fig. 7.5 Graph of J-shaped curve of response to infection.

recognize infection and to mount an appropriate antibody response.

There is a significant body of interesting research evidence to suggest that athletes in heavy training have a compromised immune response. This is widely regarded as one of the causes for athletes becoming more susceptible to minor infections at times of heavy training load. Athletes under physical and psychological stress are said to have a "J-shaped" curve of response to infection as demonstrated in Fig. 7.5.

The treatment of IM must acknowledge the natural course of this infection that may leave its legacy of lethargy for many months. While prolonged bed rest is not necessary, rest from strenuous training is strongly recommended. Coach and swimmer must understand that any attempt to "train through" the convalescent phase of this condition will simply prolong the symptoms. Pressure must come off the athlete to allow the body's natural defenses to overcome the viral invader. In some cases secondary bacterial infections are appropriately treated with antibiotics but there is no effective antiviral agent currently available to combat the EB virus. Clinical evidence for the use of intramuscular injections of vitamin B_{12} is purely anecdotal. Current symptomatic treatment of the fever and acute symptoms still provide the best long-term results. There must be agreement to allow a natural immune response to proceed without the added insult of prolonged physical stress. Once the acute symptoms have disappeared, physical activity is permitted but at a low intensity at the discretion of the swimmer. In about 70% of sufferers there is enlargement of the spleen with an attendant serious potential for rupture. Heavy physical exertion or water polo and diving are not advised during this acute phase.

Skin conditions

Exposure to a constant moist environment leaves the skin of the aquatic athlete very prone to various skin problems. These may include fungal, viral, or bacterial infections with typical features and characteristic sites of body involvement.

Fungal infections

Common sites of fungal skin infection are the spaces between the toes (interdigital spaces) and the groin region. These conditions are referred to as "athlete's foot" (tinea pedis) or "jock itch" (tinea cruris) respectively.

A skin scraping examined under UVL will demonstrate the classical presence of fungal elements confirming the diagnosis and the need for a topical antifungal agent. In cases of chronic infection involving the toe or fingernails, a longer course of oral medication may be required, under the recommendation of a specialist dermatologist. Occasionally, to relieve the annoying itch associated with fungal infection the use of corticosteroid cream may be indicated. Prevention of infection should still be the goal. Scrupulous drying between the toes, frequent changes of socks, and the use of suitable footwear in showers and on pool decks are simple measures to be encouraged.

Viral skin infections

There are two common sources of potential viral infection associated with aquatic sports. The first of these is infection by the human wart virus that is the cause of plantar warts (verrucae) and the second is the spread of herpes simplex virus (HSV) from shared towels.

Plantar warts are common on the soles of the feet where they invade the local dermis and can produce thickened, painful lesions that may become rather unsightly. To reduce the risk of transmission, swimmers should be encouraged to wear suitable footwear in the showers and generally around the pool deck precincts. Treatment options include various topical applications, the use of cryotherapy, or in some recalcitrant cases, surgical excision with electric cautery.

HSV infections, also known as "cold sores," may appear as painful blisters that erupt on the face. Commonly they occur on the lips but the risk of spread to the nose or eyes carries an added difficulty in treatment and the potential for serious complication. This virus may remain dormant for months or years to become reactivated at times of "stress," reflecting its opportunistic tendency at times of immune suppression. A closely related form of HSV is responsible for lesions of the genital tract. Antiviral creams are available to treat HSV or in acute serious cases oral medication is available that may help to control this troublesome condition. Medical advice should always be sought if HSV infection is suspected.

Bacterial infection

Competitive swimmers frequently shave their bodies to reduce drag and this habit has lead to the recognition of a particular form of skin infection known as "swimmer's folliculitis." Repetitive shaving reduces natural protective layers of skin and facilitates infection by microorganisms such as *Staphylococcus* or *Pseudomonas* species. Topical antibiotics are usually successful in clearing these infections but sometimes there is a need for oral antibiotic therapy, and this should always be on the recommendation of a physician.

Urticaria in aquatic athletes

Some open water swimmers may experience a disturbing form of skin reaction on exposure to cold water and sunlight. This is called *urticaria*, a condition that typically causes an itchy, raised "wheal" on the skin of athletes with a known allergic tendency. These skin lesions usually respond to standard antihistamine therapy taken orally or applied locally. Less-frequent cases of exercise-induced urticaria deserve to be more closely monitored and referred for medical opinion, given their potential for more serious consequences.

Overtraining in swimmers

This interesting and somewhat contentious issue has been the topic of considerable debate for many years. Attempts to clearly define "overtraining" (staleness) have eluded experts in sport science. The only point of common agreement is the fact that overtraining is a combination of physical and psychosocial factors that result in failing adaptation to the sustained stress of training and competition. While the most dramatic sign of this phenomenon is the inexplicable loss of form by the swimmer, a number of objective clinical markers have been identified. Unfortunately, though, there is no single laboratory test that will quantify overtraining or accurately predict it. Clearly the body needs time to recover from recurrent, prolonged stress and when there is insufficient recovery time overtraining may result. Overtrained swimmers may complain of insomnia, loss of appetite, mood changes, altered bowel habit, muscle soreness, and frequent, annoying, minor illnesses. On clinical examination the swimmer may have an elevated resting pulse rate, altered blood parameters, including raised muscle enzymes and distinct abnormalities in their resting electrocardiograph (ECG). It is important for any swimmer whose presentation suggests overtraining to have a full medical examination to rule out such things as chronic viral infection (IM) or anemia.

The management of the overtraining syndrome involves a clear and full explanation together with honest communication between the swimmer, coach, and physician. Having ruled out treatable clinical causes, the overtrained swimmer deserves a break from training and appropriate support. The return to regular physical activity and competition may take several months. Frequent clinical follow-up is essential to reassure both athlete and coach.

The use of performance enhancing drugs in swimming

It is not within the scope of this book to provide either a complete list of banned substances or to reproduce the full FINA Doping Rules. These matters are under continuous scrutiny and the most current lists and opinions are available on the FINA Web site. FINA has a very clear and widely publicized stance on drug misuse based on the established guidelines of the IOC and the World Anti-Doping Agency (WADA). *Doping is a violation of these rules, and all competitive swimmers must be prepared to submit to doping control both in and out of competition.*

A doping offence is deemed to have occurred if a prohibited substance is detected within a swimmer's body tissue or fluids. Likewise, the refusal to submit to doping control is also deemed an offence. Sanctions are set by FINA in accordance with an international acknowledgment of the different categories of banned substances. For example, the misuse of anabolic steroids, peptide hormones, or masking agents carries the highest level of sanctioning from a minimum of 2 years expulsion for a first offence. Lesser degrees of sanction apply to the misuse of substances such as ephedrine and caffeine. (For a full update of the FINA Doping Control Rules readers are again referred to the FINA website: www.fina.org.)

WADA has taken over the responsibility for establishing international guidelines from its headquarters in Montreal. All major International Federations (IFs) share a concern for the increasing problems associated with the misuse of drugs in sport. The education of all coaches and athletes remains the prime objective. FINA, through its Sports Medicine Committee and Doping Control Review Board, places continuing emphasis on education.

Nutritional supplements

An issue of continuing concern is the escalating use of nutritional supplements by athletes. Products in this category include a wide range of "natural" products not subjected to scientific research and frequently not accurately labeled. A number of products advertised as possessing ergogenic properties are often only substantiated by anecdotal comment in the nonscientific, lay press. Few, if any, are supported by well-controlled scientific studies.

Before considering the use of any nutritional supplement athletes should always consult an expert in medical and nutritional matters, and then ask themselves the following questions:
- Is my diet meeting the nutritional demands of my sport?
- What form of supplementation is necessary and why?
- Is this supplement safe to take?
- Does it meet legal and ethical requirements?
- Am I simply being influenced by peer pressure and manufacturers' claims?

Supplementation must never be seen as a substitute for a balanced healthy diet. Where a swimmer has a documented deficiency, such as iron, there is sound evidence for supplementation. However the athlete must accept sole responsibility for whatever they choose to take. Supplements may contain substances called "prohormones" that stimulate the production of natural hormones such as testosterone that could give rise to a positive test. If ever in doubt, swimmers should not use any form of supplementation. Sport careers have been destroyed by the indiscriminate use of supplements on very dubious clinical or scientific grounds.

There are no shortcuts to success in sport. Hard training, a sensible diet, and guidance from a good coach are the fundamental prerequisites.

Promoting performance through injury prevention, by Wayne M. Goldsmith

Injury prevention is an important part of the training plan of every coach. Because of the high repetition involved in swimming training, the injuries that are most common are of the overuse variety. Here are 10 simple tips that all coaches can use to promote performance through injury prevention.

1 *Develop a network of sports medicine/science specialists*: Get to know your local sports physiotherapist, sports MD, sports massage therapist, podiatrist, etc.

2 *Screening*: Prevention is better than cure! Have your local sports physiotherapist screen your squad for possible problems.

3 *Stretching*: Stretching is often considered to be nothing more than an activity during warm-up for injury prevention. However, stretching has an important role in performance! Increasing the range of motion of different joints will make for a more efficient swimmer.

4 *Strengthening*: One purpose of a strengthening program is to limit and reduce injuries.

5 *Technique*: Generally speaking, strokes performed with correct technique are less likely to cause injury because the movements are more efficient.

6 *Backstroke and kicking*: Backstroke has an important role in injury prevention. Using backstroke works other muscles between long fly and freestyle sets and helps reduce the load on the muscles and tendons of the shoulder. Coaches have also used kicking to reduce training stresses on shoulders and arms. It is important that swimmers using boards cross their arms on the board or do not use a board at all. Kicking with the arms straight out in front only increases the strain on the point of the shoulder . . . the very thing the kick set is supposed to be relieving!

7 *Parental education*: Parents can be the frontline in injury prevention and management strategy.

8 *Massage*: Massage is extremely useful in three forms: (1) professionally done, (2) swimmers massaging themselves, and (3) parents massaging swimmers.

9 *First aid/medical kit/ice*: An important part of every coach's responsibility is having a well-maintained and up-to-date medical kit close by at all training sessions, and at all swim meets, AND being able to administer basic first aid in case of emergency. Ice should be available at all sessions and meets as part of your injury prevention and management strategy.

10 *Coach education*: It is vital that all coaches keep up to date with current injury prevention strategies and injury management techniques.

Recommended reading

Brenner, I.K.M., Shek, P.N. & Shephard, R.J. (1994) Infection in athletes. *Sports Medicine* **17**, 86–107.

Fricker, P.A. (1997) Infectious problems in athletes: an overview. In: K. Fields & P. Fricker, eds. *Medical Problems in Athletes*. Malden, MA: Blackwell Science, pp. 3–5.

Fricker, P.A., Gleeson, M., Flanagan, A., Pyne, D.B., McDonald, W.A. & Clancy, R.L. (2000) A clinical snapshot: do elite swimmers experience more upper respiratory illness than non-athletes? *Journal of Clinical Exercise Physiology* **2**, 155–158.

Gleeson, M., McDonald, W.A., Pyne, D.B., Cripps, A.W., Francis, J.L., Fricker, P.A. & Clancy, R.L. (1999) Salivary IgA levels and infection risk in elite swimmers. *Medicine and Science in Sports and Exercise* **31**, 67–73.

Gleeson, M. & Pyne, D. (2000) Exercise effects on mucosal immunity. *Immunology and Cell Biology* **78**, 536–544.

Pyne, D., McDonald, W., Gleeson, M., Flanagan, A., Clancy, R.L. & Fricker, P.A. (2001) Mucosal immunity, respiratory illness, and competitive performance in elite swimmers. *Medicine and Science in Sports and Exercise* **33**, 348–353.

Pyne, D.B., Gleeson, M., McDonald, W.A., Clancy, R.L., Perry, C. & Fricker, P.A. (2000) Training strategies to maintain immunocompetence in athletes. *International Journal of Sports Medicine* **21**, S51–S60.

Chapter 8
Training and testing of competitive swimmers

David B. Pyne and Wayne M. Goldsmith

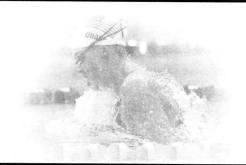

Two of the most common features of training programs of swimmers competitive are (1) the periodization of training volume and intensity and (2) the transition from training to racing. A periodized training and tapering program is based on the principle of overload–recovery–peaking. This principle forms the basis of preparing swimming training programs with the aim of increasing the level of competitive performance. A fundamental principle of preparing athletes is that periodization and tapering applies equally to all the different aspects of fitness, such as endurance, speed, strength, flexibility, and power. The training program must provide an overload (stimulus) to force the body to adapt to a previously unencountered level of stress. After sufficient application of the stimulus (in terms of magnitude and frequency), a period of recovery and regeneration will allow residual fatigue to dissipate. If the processes of overload and recovery are managed correctly a period of super compensation will occur so that performance is elevated to a higher level for important competitions.

Periodization can be defined as the division of the annual training plan into smaller and more manageable phases of training. This approach permits one aspect of fitness to be the focus of training, while maintaining the development of other aspects. In essence a periodized training program is really about being an organized and systematic coach. The transition from training to racing is commonly referred to as the taper and is characterized by a reduction in the volume of training and the development of race speed. Both periodization and the taper lead to the peaking of

performance necessary for high-level and international competition.

From a physiological viewpoint, there are several reasons for a periodized and balanced training program leading up to major competition:
- A higher training load without excessive fatigue.
- Faster recovery and regeneration.
- Maintaining performances close to their maximum for a long period of time.
- Correct peaking for the major competition of the year.
- Maintaining a basic level of fitness over a long period of training (or even a period of reduced training).
- A greater degree of specificity for individual events.
- A more efficient and effective taper (and supercompensation) process.
- More complete adaptation to training without two or three parts of the program interfering with each other when trained concurrently.
- Better planning for both major and minor competitions.
- More effective integration of sports science support with the training program.

Periodization

Periodization involves dividing the training plan into smaller parts using the terms mesocycle, macrocycle, and microcycle. These terms are used to establish a hierarchy of training within the overall program. This approach is well established in practice in a wide range of endurance and power sports.

Mesocycle

Mesocycle refers to a long-term training phase lasting several weeks to months. In swimming this represents the entire 12–20-week preparation for a major national or international competition. Most commonly, there are two mesocycles a year with peaks for the national swimming championships and then the major international competition (e.g., Olympics, Worlds, etc.) held later in the year (July–September). The length of the mesocycle will depend on the specific training and/or competition objectives for the mesocycle and the individual swimmer's current fitness level. It is apparent that coaches of leading international swimmers are incorporating more variety within the macrocycles than a few years ago.

Macrocycle

The term macrocycle refers to shorter training blocks within the mesocycle. Typically these are 2–4 weeks in length. The duration of a macrocycle depends on the objectives and type of training used in each stage of the annual plan. In physiological terms, the macrocycle is used to develop or improve a specific aspect of fitness. The classical structure of a macrocycle involves two to four "developmental" or "accumulation" microcycles (increasing volume) followed by an "intensification" or "tuning" microcycle (increasing intensity). A number of macrocycles form a single mesocycle. Experience has shown that after several weeks of intensive or extensive work, most athletes require some period of recovery (and within macrocycles as well). There are many types of macrocycle depending on the requirements of the program, coach, and athlete. Some examples used by swimming coaches are the introductory macrocycle (general training, low volume–low intensity), preparatory macrocycle (transition from low volume–low intensity to higher volume training), specific macrocycle (more specialized higher intensity training, with emphasis on improving competitive speed), and the competition macrocycle (competitive performance on a single or repeated basis). In each case, the volume and intensity of work will vary according to the specific requirements of the program and individual athlete. The better coaches

(and swimmers) are always aware of "where they are up to" in the training program. Losing speed and experiencing excessive fatigue and staleness in long and arduous meso- or macro-cycles is not a very efficient approach to training. Athletes should not struggle with their training for more than a few days without some intervention.

Microcycle

The term microcycle refers to a short-term training block within a macrocycle. The aim of the microcycle is to target specific components of fitness. Most commonly swimming training microcycles are planned around a standard 7-day training week. Coaches and athletes are creatures of the modern working week and most swimmers have to fit their training programs around work, education, and family commitments. However, coming in to important meets such as the Olympics, the training schedule takes precedence and the day of the week, weekends, and public holidays become less important. The microcycles represent the specific plans and strategies needed to achieve the broader objective of the macrocycle. The microcycle consists of the individual (daily) workouts based on the objectives of the macrocycle.

Volume before intensity

One of the fundamental principles that underpins the periodization of training is that volume of training is increased before the intensity of training. This principle applies to meso-, macro-, and microcycles alike. Most coaches are familiar with the concept that a foundation of aerobic fitness is established early in the mesocycle or competition season. After this initial period of increasing training volume to build endurance, the emphasis of training switches to the development of speed and anaerobic capacities. It is often observed that this base level of fitness can be reestablished fairly quickly (4–6 weeks) in those swimmers with an extensive training background. This has implications for older more mature swimmers who are returning after a break from training or competition. However, it is much more efficient for swimmers to maintain a basic fitness program during the off-season. A reasonable level of fitness can be maintained on about 30% of the full training volume, i.e., a swimmer who normally undertakes 10 training sessions per week, should be able to maintain a base level of fitness for several weeks by just training three times per week. In this case, it is important to maintain some intensity in the work (up to and including threshold level) when volume and duration are reduced.

This principle of volume first, then intensity, also applies to strength and muscular endurance. In a fashion similar to that for endurance training, strength programs are often based on an initial period of volume training (lighter weight–many repetitions) before more intensive training (heavier weight–fewer repetitions) is undertaken. On this basis, a typical 4-week strength program (e.g., free weights, machine weights, circuits) for endurance athletes takes the form of a 2-week macrocycle of volume training and then a 2-week cycle of intensity training. While some coaches and swimmers place a heavy emphasis on strength training, it is clear that strength alone is not highly correlated with swimming performance. Other factors like muscular power, muscular endurance and muscle elasticity, and of course, swimming technique, should not be overlooked.

In terms of designing microcycles the "volume first, intensity second" principle is also valuable. One approach that we have found to be successful is the use of 3-day microcycles. A detailed example of a 3-day microcycle is presented later in this chapter (Table 8.4). The first variant involves two training sessions a day for the first 2 days, followed by a single session on the third day. In some circumstances in swimming, where three training sessions a day are used, the second variation takes the form of three sessions a day for 2 days and then two sessions on the third and final day. In both versions, the first day is largely aerobic in nature, with a gradual decrease in volume and increase in intensity as the microcycle proceeds. The emphasis is on increasing speed from day to day, and athletes generally find this easier if the training volume is decreasing. Many swimmers (and coaches) like to finish each microcycle with a quality or speed session.

Another feature of planning is the relationship between duration and intensity. Generally speaking, the lower the intensity of cycles, the longer the duration, perhaps up to 7 days. For higher intensity work, shorter 2–4 day training cycles are used. Variation of training distance and intensity within cycles is important. Early in the program, microcycles may involve higher intensity training for athletes already fatigued. The thinking is that this approach provides a greater stimulus for adaptation. Later on, when the emphasis is on competition-specific speed, it is usually better to undertake high-intensity training in a fresh condition in order to facilitate higher speeds.

Training plan for a season

The contemporary model of preparing competitive swimmers in a given year is based on the following sequence of training and competition: preseason, early season, competitive season, taper, championship season, and recovery or off-season. For highly trained swimmers the competitive season usually takes the form of domestic competition or international competitions like the FINA World Cup Series. The championship season typically involves the national championships, often doubling as the national team selection trials, and then the major international competition for that particular year.

Once the competition schedule has been established, the training plan can be prepared with the goal of maximizing the performance of the swimmer for the competitive and championship seasons. For international swimmers, the entire season is typically 44–48 weeks in length with a short break permitted after completion of the championship season. The length of each of the different training phases will vary according to the individual circumstances of the swimmer, team, and coach. In recent years, the international swimming calendar has become more crowded and as a consequence the annual training plan has become more fragmented and complex. A common view of experienced coaches is that this trend has been beneficial for sprint swimming, but detrimental to distance swimming. The relative plateauing of world records in women's distance swimming provides some support for this view.

The evolution of the modern training plan can be viewed from three perspectives. The traditional approach to the annual plan and individual training sessions has centered on the different energy systems as they apply to competitive swimming. The three energy systems model has enjoyed great popularity in coach education, but its relevance for the practicing coach is somewhat limited. Clearly there are many other factors, apart from the proportional contribution from each of the three energy systems, that need to be considered. To address some of these long-standing concerns a new approach that integrates physiological, biomechanical, and psychological aspects of exercise and training has been proposed (Noakes 2000). Irrespective of the conceptual framework, coaches and swimmers are primarily interested in the prescription of training velocities. The most appropriate means of prescribing training velocities is achieved through evaluation of the competitive model that identifies the performance requirements of each individual event (Mason 1999).

Prescription of training speeds

Training by competitive swimmers typically consists of repeated bouts of shorter or longer intervals in a short-course or long-course pool. Intervals span a continuum from longer slower intervals (50–1600 m for developing aerobic or endurance fitness) to shorter faster intervals (15–200 m for developing anaerobic or race pace qualities). The basic prescription of interval training can be simplified to four primary variables: (i) the number of intervals or repeat efforts, (ii) the length/distance of the interval (15 m to continuous swimming), (iii) the intensity (i.e., pace or velocity) of the interval, and (iv) the rest period between intervals (variously formulated as the cycle time or rest period). The resulting training sets can be presented in the well established format of number of

intervals/repeats × distance (pace) on cycle time/rest period. Two examples are 20 × 100 m (1:20) on 2:00, and 16 × 50 m (@ 200 m race pace) on 1:30.

A fundamental challenge for coaches and scientists is the accurate determination of specific training paces. A common approach is to base training times on the goal or predicted competition time for each individual swimmer. At the international level, this is achieved by examination of the most recent championship performances and where necessary forward projection to the upcoming major competition. To illustrate this process, the winning time for each gold medalist in the freestyle and form stroke events at the Sydney 2000 Olympic Games is shown in Table 8.1. It is interesting to note differences in performance time between distances (in the freestyle events), between events (in the form strokes), and between male and female swimmers. The average pace per 100 m provides a mean of comparing the pace of different events in a format commonly used by coaches. The percentage difference in average pace from the 50 m to the 1500-m freestyle at the 2000 Olympic Games was approximately 27%. This variation in pace provides a substantial challenge for coaches with large training squads comprising swimmers of different sexes, levels, strokes, and distances.

Preseason

Preseason training commences from the low base of fitness maintained during the off-season. Swimmers typically start the preseason phase with a single session per day and gradually increase the number of sessions over the first few weeks. A graded increase sees

Table 8.1 Comparison of performance times and swimming paces in male and female gold medallists (selected events) at the Sydney 2000 Olympic Games.

| | | Event (m) | | | | | | | | | | | |
| | | FS | | | | | | Fly | | BK | | BR | |
		50	100	200	400	800	1500	100	200	100	200	100	200
Male	Time	21.9	48.3	1.45.3	3.40.6	–	14.48.3	52.0	1.55.4	53.7	1.56.8	60.5	2.10.9
	s/100 m	43.8	48.3	52.7	55.2	–	59.2	52.0	57.7	53.7	58.4	60.5	65.5
Female	Time	24.3	53.8	1.58.2	4.05.8	8.19.7	–	56.6	2.05.9	60.2	2.08.2	67.1	2.24.4
	s/100 m	48.6	53.8	59.1	61.5	62.5		56.6	62.9	60.2	64.1	67.1	72.2

Performances are presented in both absolute (performance time) and relative (pace expressed as s/100 m) terms for ease of comparison. FS: freestyle; Fly: butterfly; BK: backstroke; BR: breaststroke.

the frequency of training increasing from one session per day, to three sessions over 2 days, and eventually to the traditional two sessions per day format followed by the majority of high-level swimmers. The intensity of swimming is low to moderate to facilitate structural improvements leading toward improved cardiorespiratory fitness. Slower swimming also permits the acquisition and development of skills at lower speeds, before transfer to faster competitive speeds. A limited amount of shorter faster work is recommended, even from the first week of the season, to develop and maintain neuromuscular patterns. This approach prepares the swimmer for the more intensive training that follows in the early-season and competitive-season phases.

Early season

The main features of the early-season phase are a modest training volume to start, small 5–10 km increases in volume per week, low initial training intensity, and dry-land conditioning including flexibility, circuits, weight training, and other games and activities, to improve the overall sport abilities of the swimmer. After several weeks there are further increases in training volume, a gradual introduction of higher intensity aerobic work to the level of the lactate threshold, and emphasis on skill and technique development before moving to the faster training speeds. In simple terms, training volume elicits improvements in general endurance fitness while training intensity develops the specific fitness required for racing and competitive success. The later weeks of the early-season phase focus on continuing development of the lactate threshold (endurance fitness), maximal oxygen uptake (maximal aerobic) and race pace training capacities, ongoing manipulation of training volume and intensity to maintain improvement, an individualized approach to volume, intensity and recovery, and refinement of skills particularly at race speeds.

The early-season phase is based on sequential increases in the volume and intensity of training. The prescription of swimming training in its simplest form is achieved by manipulation of these two factors. Training volume in swimming is relatively easy to quantify, and forms the basis of most modern swimming programs. Multiples of laps are easily added to determine the total distance covered in a single set,

session, or training week. Most coaches and swimmers are comfortable with the notion and terminology relating, for example, to a 2000-m set (e.g. 20×100 m), a 6000-m session or a 40-km week. High-level training involving planning for the longer period (e.g., the annual plan or even the 4 year Olympic quadrennium) necessitates the calculation of long-term training volumes. For example, coaches can plan for a 2-week training camp (e.g., 140 km in a 14-day camp), a complete preparation or training macrocycle (e.g., 500 km for a 12-week cycle), or a full training year (e.g., 2000 km in 46 weeks). Although these calculations can be time consuming they are useful in the planning and review of coaching programs.

A central issue in planning relates to the relative potency (and paradoxically, the relative danger) of substantial increases in training volume and intensity. Although high training volumes, and periodic doses of high-intensity training, are a fundamental part of training, the problems associated with excessive training, particularly when coupled with inadequate recovery, are known to all coaches. Coaching experience and the results of scientific research collectively suggest that excessive training volume and training intensity can induce fatigue, overtraining, injury, or illness. Coaches are aware that distance swimmers generally require higher training volumes (approximately 20–25% more than sprint swimmers) to develop the background necessary for success in events ranging from the 400 to 1500 m. In practice, substantial increases in either training volume or intensity during the early season places considerable physical demands and stress on the body. Some swimmers exhibit fatigue and poor performance when training loads are excessively high and recovery is incomplete, although this state is largely reversible with a few days rest.

In contrast to training volume, training intensity is more difficult to quantify. A systematic approach is required for effective planning and monitoring of training intensity. The most common approach involves the use of a training classification system that gives rise to different training intensities. In the past the majority of these training systems have relied on relatively subjective descriptors of intensity. This practice has given rise to a wide range of terminology (e.g., moderate intensity aerobic, aerobic threshold, anaerobic threshold, lactate tolerance, onset of blood

Table 8.2 Training classification system used at the Australian Institute of Sport showing different intensity coefficients.

Zone	Symbol	Fuel	Intensity (%)	HR (bpm)	La (mm)	Intensity coefficient
Low-intensity aerobic	A1	Fat	65–75	−70 to −50	< 2	1
Aerobic maintenance	A2	Fat/CHO	75–80	−40 to −50	< 2	1
Aerobic development	A3	Fat/CHO	80–85	−30 to −40	2–3	2
Lactate threshold	LT	Fat/CHO	85–92	−20 to −30	3–5	3
Maximal aerobic	MVO_2	CHO	92–100	−20 to max	5–10	5
Sprint	SP	ATP-PC	> 100	n/a	n/a	8

HR: heart rate; La: lactate; CHO: carbohydrate; ATP-PC: adenosine triphosphate phosphocreatine.

lactate accumulation, maximal alactic anaerobic) that is difficult to distinguish in practice (Counsilman & Counsilman 1993). To overcome the problems of terminology and to provide a more quantitative basis, scientists have devised various systems where different intensities of swimming are ascribed a particular "weighting or physiological stress coefficient" (Mujika et al. 1996). This process is based on the blood lactate concentration that presumably reflects the physiological demand of different exercise intensities.

To illustrate this approach, the training classification system devised for swimmers at the Australian Institute of Sport is shown in Table 8.2. The most important feature is that the degree of physiological stress experienced by the swimmer increases exponentially above the level of the lactate threshold. Proportionally greater weighting coefficients are given to the higher training intensity levels. Low- and moderate-intensity aerobic efforts have the lowest weighting coefficients, while the more intensive maximal aerobic training is given a proportionally higher coefficient. Sprint training (which can be the most physiologically demanding) is given the highest coefficient. Other modeling systems employ a similar system of weighting coefficients. This type of approach to monitoring training intensity has given rise to the development of additional descriptors of training such as training load (the product of training volume and training intensity), training monotony, and training strain (the product of training load and monotony) (Foster 1998).

Tapering

The tapering strategy used by many swimmers to optimize competition performance has been defined as "a progressive non-linear reduction of the training load during a variable period of time, in an attempt to reduce the physiological and psychological stress of daily training and optimize sports performance" (Mujika & Padilla 2000). The aim of the taper before the main competitions of the season is to elicit substantial improvements in performance. These performance gains have been variously attributed to increased levels of muscular force and power (Trappe et al. 2000), and improvements in neuromuscular, hematological, and hormonal function, and/or the psychological status of the swimmer (Mujika & Padilla 2000). The main features of the taper include a systematic 3–4 week reduction in training volume, ongoing aerobic work to maintain basic fitness and develop race fitness, and fine tuning of race pace and pacing strategies through use of descending sets, broken swims, and time trials. Training volume is gradually reduced reaching about 20% of the peak weekly mileage at the time of competition. The conventional wisdom in the swimming community holds that male and sprint swimmers generally require a longer taper than female and distance swimmers respectively.

A study of the taper of swimmers competing at the 2000 Olympic Games revealed a mean performance improvement of $2.2 \pm 1.5\%$ (range −1.1 to 6.0%) over the final 3 weeks of training (Mujika et al. 2002). A total of 91 out of the 99 analyzed performances were faster at the Olympic Games after the taper and only 8 were slower. The percentage improvement in performance time was greater in the males ($2.6 \pm 1.5\%$) (mean ± standard deviation) than the females ($1.8 \pm 1.5\%$). The improvement of ~2% in performance with the taper similar for all Olympic events and was achieved by swimmers from different countries and performance levels. This information provides a quantitative framework for coaches and swimmers to set realistic performance goals based on individual performance levels.

Championship season

The championship season is all about competitive performance rather than responses to training. Estimates of progression and variability of performance in competitions are useful for coaches, swimmers, and researchers interested in factors affecting performance (Hopkins *et al.* 1999; Trewin *et al.* 2004). Progressions are generally required to ensure that a swimmer qualifies for the semifinal and then the final in a given event, and that peak performance is produced in the final, where medals are decided. Performance evaluations of this type for leading swimmers provide some insight into the variability and progression of performance of both individuals and teams (Stewart & Hopkins 2000). This information also assists swimmers and coaches in the planning process.

The utility of these estimates was examined in swimmers of the world's top two swimming nations competing in the 2000 Olympic Games (Pyne *et al.* in press). Official race times ($n = 676$) of 26 US and 25 Australian Olympic swimmers who competed in the 1999 Pan Pacific Championships, the 2000 Olympic Trials, and the 2000 Olympic Games were analyzed. Within each competition, both nations showed similar improvements of 1.2% in mean performance time from heats through finals. Mean competition time improved in the 12 months between the Pan Pacifics and Olympics by approximately 0.9%. The typical variation in performance time for a swimmer between races was 0.6% within a competition and 0.8% between competitions. Sex and swimming distance appeared to have minor or negligible effects on progression and variability. These findings suggest that an Olympic swimmer has to improve performance by ∼1% within a competition to stay in contention for a medal and by ∼1% within the year leading to the Olympics.

The variation in performance from race to race is an important determinant of a swimmer's chances of winning the race. A swimmer in contention for a medal has to improve his or her performance by approximately half the typical race-to-race variation in performance (expressed as a standard deviation) to substantially increase their chance of success. However, other swimmers may also improve their performance between competitions, so a given swimmer will need to improve by an additional amount approximately equal to the mean progression of all

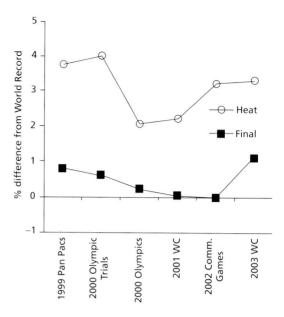

Fig. 8.1 Progression in performance time of Ian Thorpe in the men's 400-m freestyle over a 4-year period from the 1999 Pan Pacs to the 2003 World Championships (WC). Heat and final shown for each meet. Data are expressed as percentage difference from the world record swim at the 2002 Commonwealth Games.

the competitors to remain in contention. An example of progressions in performance time for the 2000 Olympic and 2001 and 2003 World Champion Ian Thorpe (Australia) in the 400-m freestyle is shown in Fig. 8.1 and Table 8.3.

Recovery or off-season

The main features of this phase are maintaining an active approach with at least three low- to moderate-intensity aerobic swims completed each week, specialized programs to target weaknesses in individual fitness profiles, and dietary control to maintain body composition. There are few studies that have directly addressed the issue of the most effective program for swimmers to follow during the off-season or in short breaks from training and competition. There is, however, a significant body of literature that details the time course of training adaptations with training and loss of fitness during detraining (Counsilman & Counsilman 1991; Mujika & Padilla 2000). A typical strategy for the off-season involves a marked 50–70% reduction in the frequency, volume, and intensity of training.

Table 8.3 Progression in 400-m freestyle performance time in heats and finals over a 4-year period for Ian Thorpe (Australia), the World Record Holder, World Championships, and Olympic Gold Medalist.

Meet	Heat	Final
1999 Pan Pacs	3.48.36	3.41.83
2000 Olympic Trials	3.48.93	3.41.43
2000 Olympic Games	3.44.65	3.40.59
2001 World Championships	3.45.02	3.40.17
2002 Commonwealth Games	3.47.24	3.40.08
2003 World Championships	3.47.44	3.42.58
Mean	3.46.94	3.41.11
SD	1.7	1.0
%CV	0.8	0.5

All Final swims were world records except for the 2003 World Championships.
CV: coefficient of variation = mean/SD; SD: standard deviation

For a highly trained swimmer, who normally completes 10 training sessions per week, this would equate to approximately three sessions of low- to moderate-intensity training. Apart from maintaining the underlying cardiovascular and metabolic adaptations, regular training will also help retain neuromuscular patterns and the all important "feel for the water."

Periodizing to build endurance and speed—An example

The following is an example of the features of periodization that may encompass a typical 14-week swimming preparation for a national championships or major international meet.

Macrocycle 1: aerobic (weeks 1–4)

As in most training programs the initial phase involves the development or reestablishment of endurance fitness. This serves as the basis for the subsequent development of aerobic and anaerobic capacities and the functional utilization of these capacities. Functional utilization refers to increased swimming speed at a given metabolic load. Apart from the underlying physiological adaptations, improved endurance will lead to an increased ability to cope with fatigue and more rapid recovery from the stresses of speed training and competition. In particular, the aim is to develop the capacity and efficiency of the cardiorespiratory system. This process is largely achieved by high volume–low intensity training. Other adaptations include increased utilization of fat as a fuel source, stronger ligaments, tendons and connective tissue, adaptations within slow-twitch muscle fibers, and improved neuromuscular control. The length of this phase will depend on several factors (e.g., fitness level of athletes, time available, objectives of mesocycle) but is normally between 3–4 weeks.

Macrocycle 2: aerobic/anaerobic (weeks 5–8)

In this macrocycle, the other primary components of aerobic training are developed. Assuming that low to moderate intensity endurance work is developed in the first microcycle, this cycle is characterized by an emphasis on lactate threshold training. For example, the 200 m swimmers undertake up to 30% of work in this cycle at the level of lactate threshold, and up to 15% of maximal oxygen uptake and lactate tolerance work. Some coaches may think these levels are too low for middle-distance and sprint athletes (the levels will vary for different sports and events). The total training volume is increased over macrocycle 1 and there is a progressive introduction of shorter and faster intervals. The duration of the macrocycle is normally 2–3 weeks.

Macrocycle 3: transition (weeks 9–12)

In many ways this is the key training phase. The aim is to develop the functional utilization of the energy systems and capacities that were established in the aerobic endurance and aerobic/anaerobic macrocycles. It is well documented that the factor that correlates most highly with endurance performance is the speed at lactate threshold. This is an important point that is often overlooked. To illustrate this point consider the following example: Swimmer A is likely to perform better if his or her speed is faster than swimmer B at the same relative lactate threshold. Improving the functional utilization (speed at a given metabolic load) is achieved through training drills of higher intensity but shorter duration, at speeds close to and faster than competitive speeds. The high degree of aerobic fitness developed earlier will be maintained even though the emphasis of training is on higher quality intervals. This macrocycle is fairly short with an average length of 3–4 weeks.

Macrocycle 4: taper and competition (weeks 12–14)

The final macrocycle within the season (mesocycle) involves the taper period and the competition phase. Again the logic follows the preceding macrocycle and training is characterized by a further reduction in training volume, and the development of speed and power. In swimming, it is common to reduce the training volume by approximately half (50%) to two thirds (67%) of the peak weekly volume for the preparation. The key is to reduce the volume and sharpen the speed. This process involves shorter intervals at faster than race pace, e.g., for 100-m swimmers there would be an emphasis on 25 and 50-m intervals at faster than 100 m race pace. It is important to maintain some aerobic training in this macrocycle and a common mistake is to reduce training mileage too rapidly. Aerobic work is needed to support the taper and forms an essential part of the recovery and regeneration process prior to competition.

Coaching tips, by Wayne M. Goldsmith

1 The most important consideration is that peaking for performance is an active process. Put as much effort into the planning and execution of the tapering and peaking program as you do for regular training.

2 The annual plan and the competition calendar are essential tools. To achieve extraordinary results you need an extraordinarily good training program. Last year's program may bring you last year's results.

3 Make sure your athletes are able to train at close to race speed when required. This is achieved by careful management of endurance, speed, and recovery.

4 Plan broad details for a mesocycle, fine details for a microcycle, and adjust details on a daily basis.

5 Although the requirement for aerobic work applies to the middle distance and distance events, even the shorter sprint events may benefit from this type of training.

6 A more effective approach is to have a broad-based conditioning program. Too much concentration in one area, e.g., weight training, and neglect of others, e.g., flexibility or cross training, may be a limiting factor.

7 Be proactive: make and dictate the move from volume to intensity, endurance to speed, and training to racing.

8 When peaking, the development of race speed should take priority over conditioning work.

9 Control the intensity of training by speed (pacing), heart rate, and perception of effort (by the athlete and coach)—don't neglect any one factor.

10 Use speed-assisted drills: speed-assist device (stretch cords) or pace work with similar or faster athletes.

11 The key of peaking is to reduce volume and sharpen speed. Peaking is an active process of training, achieved by a well-planned, well-executed training and recovery program.

Sequential loading of training microcycles

This section addresses some of ways to plan a short training microcycle for competitive swimmers. A creative approach to the planning of training sessions is essential to maintain an adequate adaptation stimulus. Once the various cycles are organized within the season or yearly plan, the detailing of individual training sessions can begin.

Some coaches make the mistake of not properly integrating speed and endurance in the training program. This is particularly evident in the endurance phase where too great an emphasis on the volume of training may impair speed. It is an oversimplification to think that only low to moderate intensity volume work is undertaken in an "endurance" week or phase, and that only speed work is done in a "speed" week. If insufficient speed work is undertaken during the endurance phase, a swimmer may pay the price later on when they are unable to reproduce race or competitive speeds. Conversely, swimmers may become overloaded and prone to fatigue, illness, and injury if they do too much speed work without the benefits of some complementary endurance training. Highly trained swimmers can use endurance training to recover from and prepare for speed training.

Table 8.4 An example from the AIS Swimming Program showing the loading of an intensive 3-day microcycle. Only the main training set(s) are shown for each session. Intervals are in meters on the indicated cycle time (min:s).

	Monday	Tuesday	Wednesday
AM	8 × 400 on 5:30 [1] 5.0 (km)	1 × 1000 on 14:00 [1] 2 × 800 on 11:00 [1] 5.0 (km)	4 × 400 on 5:30 [1] 4 × 100 on 1:40 [2] 4 × 25 on 1:00 [5] 4.0 (km)
Noon	8 × 200 on 2:45 [1] 8 × 100 on 1:40 [2] 6.0 (km)	6 × 150 on 2:15 [1] 6 × 150 on 2:15 [2] 6 × 100 on 2:30 [3] 6.0 (km)	4 × 2 × 100 on 1:40 [2] 4 × 2 × 100 on 2:30 [3] 4 × 2 × 50 on 1:00 [4] 5.0 (km)
PM	4 × 200 on 2:45 [1] 4 × 100 on 1:40 [2] 4 × 2 × 25 on 1:00 [5] 3.5 (km)	4 × 400 on 6:00 [1] 4 × 25 on 1:00 [5] 3.5 (km)	Off

Intensity ratings are as follows: [1] aerobic, [2] lactate threshold, [3] maximal aerobic, [4] lactate tolerance, and [5] short sprints. Total session volumes are shown in kilometers.

Three-day microcycle example

What are some approaches to loading microcycles in swimming? One method used by the Swimming Program at the Australian Institute of Sport is to systematically increase the intensity of workouts during a 3-day microcycle. The example described here is taken from a relatively intense microcycle used to target specific areas of aerobic fitness in highly trained swimmers (Table 8.4). The basic variables of interval training (e.g., intensity, volume, duration, and frequency) are manipulated to meet the goals of each individual session and microcycle. This microcycle is for senior swimmers in good condition and may not be appropriate for age group swimmers or those returning from a layoff, injury, or illness.

Inspection of this sequence shows that the speed of training is increased systematically within each day and also across successive days (Table 8.4). Training three sessions a day is a big commitment but the benefits gained can be substantial. Apart from having the opportunity to undertake a larger volume of training, there is scope to incorporate all the important elements of training. This may simply involve working all the different strokes, drills, and sets. It also gives the opportunity for some creative coaching, like switching sets for individual medley, combination sets of varying distances and intensities, and trying out some new technique drills. One of the main benefits of three sessions a day is to improve the swimmer's feel of the water with more frequent exposure than is normally experienced. Three sessions a day is not new

and has been used occasionally by leading coaches and swimmers.

Day 1

On Day 1, aerobic intervals and some short sprints are undertaken for a total volume of 14.5 km (5.0 + 6.0 + 3.5). The AM session contains some 400s at an aerobic level. This work forms the basis of a highly trained swimmer's program, but some swimmers shy away from this type of work. Even sprinters should be prepared to undertake some basic endurance work. The main set of the Noon session is 8 × (200 on 2:45 [1], 100 on 1:40 [2]). (*Numbers in square brackets represent intensity ratings; see Table 8.4 for description of intensity ratings.*) These cycles are for freestyle and would need to be adjusted for the form strokes. Most coaches use the approach seen here of 200s at an aerobic speed and then 100s at a slightly faster threshold speed. The shorter session in the PM contains the speed work (4 × 2 × 25 m at [5]). Again the emphasis is on increasing speed as the set progresses. Swimmers should always be able to perform fast 25s even during high volume training weeks.

Day 2

On Day 2 the same training volume as on Day 1 (14.5 km) is completed but there is more quality in the Noon session. The AM session is used to prepare the swimmers for higher quality swimming in the Noon and PM sessions. The AM session has some 800s and 1000s. These are often but not always done freestyle. Mixing or alternating freestyle with freestyle/backstroke by 50-, 100-, or 200-m intervals or even individual medley in normal order or reverse order is commonly seen. A good practice is to mix up these longer intervals: some should be done straight freestyle and some using a mixed approach. Many coaches and swimmers fall into the habit of doing all the work using a mixture of strokes and distances and may miss the benefits of continuous over distance freestyle swimming. There are some programs at both senior and age-group levels that do not use these longer intervals at all—this may be limiting in the long term.

The Noon session of 6 × (150 on 2:15 at [1], 150 on 2:15 at [2], 100 on 2:30 at [3]) is a useful way to introduce more quality and speed into the workouts. This is a descending set with the first 150 swum at level [1] or aerobic, the second 150 at level [2] or threshold, and the final 100 at level [3] or maximal aerobic (approximately 400 m race pace). The final 100 is on a longer cycle time (2:30) to permit some recovery before the set is repeated. This is an example of a combination set that mixes different distances and different intensities. The total distance of the set is 2400 m, which represents a solid training session for aerobic fitness. This type of work can be used in conjunction with the commonly used "heart rate" sets, which are characterized by the repetition of the same distance at equivalent or increasing intensity, e.g., 30 × 100 m on 1:40 holding 1:05 or heart rate 160—190 bpm (40–10 beats below a maximum heart rate of 200 bpm). A commonly asked question by coaches is whether it is better to hold swimmers at a high heart rate and let their repeat times slip a little, or back them off to keep their heart rate under control. The most important thing is to maintain speed together with proper technique—if this means increasing the rest period or cycle time, or slowing the swimmer a little. There is no single answer here and a coach has to exercise his or her judgment as to the most appropriate action on the day.

Day 3

On Day 3, there are only two sessions for a total of 9 km. This gives the swimmers a better opportunity to attack the main Noon session. The aim here is to reduce the volume of training and concentrate on the

speed (intensity). Note again how the AM session contains a small build-up of intensity [1–2] to prepare the swimmers for the demanding [2–3–4] Noon session. Contrast this to the AM sessions in Days 1 and 2 where only aerobic [1] work was undertaken. Using the first session to prepare a swimmer for the second session is possible where the sessions are close together and only a few hours apart.

The final Noon session of this 3-day microcycle is 4 × (2 × 100 on 1:40 [2], 2 × 100 on 2:30 [3], and 2 × 50 on 1:00 [4]). This is the most intensive session of the microcycle both in terms of effort and speed. Note that the second pair of 2 × 100 is on a longer cycle (2:30) than the first pair (1:40). The extra time is designed to support the increase in speed, i.e., 2 × 100 on 2:30 at [3] compared with 2 × 100 on 1:40 at [2]. It is expected that the 50s would be quite fast, at around 100 m race pace. Again these cycles are for freestyle and may need to be adjusted for other strokes or junior swimmers.

Summary

This is an example of "loading volume first, then quality" within a 3-day microcycle. While most coaches are familiar with planning interval training workouts, the fundamental step involves integrating a whole sequence of interval sessions that contribute to the specific goals for that training cycle. The example presented here was a 3-day training cycle with a total of 36 km. Senior swimmers have used this type of training in high volume camps, at altitude, and in various stages of the training cycle, where the coach is looking to develop the level of aerobic fitness. Even age-group swimmers could undertake a modified version of this three sessions a day training plan during organized camps or the school holiday period. The principles and workouts discussed here are, of course, equally relevant to the more routine practice of two sessions a day.

Physiological testing of swimmers

Rationale for testing

Several benefits can be obtained from a well-organized and executed fitness-testing program. The primary objective of physiological testing is to quantify or assess various components in the fitness profile of the swimmer. A testing program monitors changes in the fitness profile at strategic points from the early-season phase through to the championship season. A second aim of testing is to determine individualized training speeds, particularly for aerobic training. A large number of testing protocols and mathematical methods (Bishop *et al.* 1998) have been derived for estimating training speeds. The so-called anaerobic or lactate threshold has been the focus of a large number of studies examining its suitability for the prescription of training speeds (Weltman 1993). Talent identification and development programs rely substantially on physiological testing to identify those individuals with the requisite anthropometric characteristics and fitness levels. Physiological testing can also be used to assess the impact of various training interventions (e.g., training methodologies, skills and drills, altitude training, strength training), dietary modifications such as manipulation of total caloric intake, macronutrients (i.e., carbohydrate, fat, and protein), and micronutrients (e.g., vitamin and minerals), and new equipment and technology (e.g., full body swimsuits) on swimming performance.

Pool-based testing

The traditional approach to the physiological assessment of competitive swimmers has centered on pool-based testing of aerobic or endurance fitness. These tests have generally used protocols involving a progressive incremental series of swims culminating in a maximal effort. Pioneering work in the metabolic assessment (oxygen uptake) of swimmers conducted in the 1970s and 1980s paved the way for a more rigorous approach to training based on physiological and metabolic parameters (Troup 1999). Logistical difficulties associated with collection of expired ventilation, and concerns over the validity of measurement techniques such as backward extrapolation (Sleivert & Mackinnon 1991), have focused attention on indirect measures of energy cost such as heart rate and blood lactate.

Observational monitoring of heart rate and blood lactate during training and competition has been a feature of international swimming in recent years. The development of portable semiautomated blood lactate analyzers in the 1980s and 1990s generated considerable interest in the swimming community (Prins 1988). A key consideration with heart rate and blood lactate testing is that physiological responses should be interpreted in the context of performance times. From a coaching perspective, the quality of a particular training set is determined by inspection of the mean time for each set of intervals, the fastest time, range of times, split times, and comparison with the respective goal or target times for the set, as well the physiological measures of heart rate and lactate. Self-reported measures of psychophysiological status such as the Borg Scale (RPE, rating of perceived exertion) are useful in monitoring the feedback of swimmers during prolonged and/or intensive training sets. In combination with physiological measures, such as blood lactate concentration, the rating of perceived exertion is a useful indicator of the presence of fatigue (Snyder *et al.* 1993).

Assessment of sprint capabilities requires testing protocols with shorter, faster intervals of 25, 50, or 100 m. Performance time and stroke mechanics (e.g., stroke rate, stroke length, stroke count) are measured. In this context, these characteristics are more important than the traditional physiological indicators of heart rate and blood lactate concentration. Swimming velocity is the product of stroke length (m/stroke) and stroke frequency (stroke rate), while the derived index of stroke efficiency is calculated as the product of stroke length (m) and swimming velocity ($m \cdot s^{-1}$). The stroke characteristics are plotted as a linear or polynomial function of swimming velocity (Pyne *et al.* 2000). Many coaches simply use a timed dive 25 m maximal effort swim to indicate the progress in developing race speed for the sprint events.

Body composition

The development and maintenance of lean body mass is an important factor in swimming where characteristics of endurance, power, and strength are associated with performance. The most common method for the assessment of body composition in elite swimmers is measurement of skinfold thickness. Despite the relative ease of simple body composition measurements, there are very few published reports on seasonal and long-term changes in competitive swimmers. There is only limited information on morphological changes (i.e., body mass, lean muscle mass, fat mass) occurring over extended periods of swimming training. Much of the information collected on competitive swimmers has been retained in individual records and not published for reasons of confidentiality, or to protect the hard-earned competitive advantage over opposition swimmers and nations.

One case study of two male swimmers reported a variable pattern of responses with one athlete losing both lean body mass and body fat, while the other increased lean mass with a reduction in subcutaneous adipose tissue (Hawes & Sovak 1994). A study of 15 elite female swimmers monitored at three points during a competitive season reported major changes during the early part of the season, with no further changes occurring during the second half of the season (Meleski & Malina 1985). There were significant losses in body fat but gains in lean body mass with training. Both of these studies produced results that are in line with the expectation of improved body composition after a successful training program. More detailed information on systematic changes in body composition through each phase of training in a given preparation, and over an athlete's career, would be a great assistance for coaches and practitioners.

Performance analysis

Performance analysis represents a new approach in swimming that links directly the results of physiological and biomechanical testing with the competitive performance of individual swimmers. Performance analysis can be categorized into two areas: (i) overall performance analysis and (ii) competitive or race modeling. Performance analysis involves monitoring the overall progression of total race times within and between competitions (Table 8.3). Progressions are generally required within a single competition to ensure that a swimmer qualifies for the semifinal and final. In the same way, progressions in training times, either in routine training sets repeated on a regular basis through the season or with standardized physiological testing, will indicate the degree of improvement or progress with training. Race modeling involves filming of swimming races and measurement of a range of performance and stroke characteristics including start time, turn

times, split times, stroke rate, stroke length, stroke efficiency, and finish time (Mason 1999). This information on a given swimmer can be compared with previous races (individual comparison), with other swimmers in the same race (group comparison), or against benchmarks such as the world record in that event (Table 8.5). Most of the major international championships since the mid 1990s have provided this information for coaches and swimmers (Table 8.6).

Competition analysis, by Wayne M. Goldsmith

Over the past 10 years, the factors that contribute to swimming successfully at top national and international competitions have been analyzed by leading sports scientists such as Dr Bruce Mason of the Australian Institute of Sport. Competition analysis breaks down racing into its various components.

- *Start time*: The first 15 m (from the starting signal to the time the swimmer's head crosses the 15-m mark from the starting wall).
- *Turn time*: A distance of 7.5 min and out of the wall (taken from the point where the swimmer's head passes through a point 7.5 m from the wall into a turn and continues until the swimmer's head passes through the same point 7.5 m from the wall on the way out of the turn).
- *Finish time*: The final 5 m (from the time the swimmer's head passes the 5 m mark from the finish wall to the actual hand touch on the wall).
- *Stroke length*: The distance the swimmer's head moves during a complete arm cycle (i.e., from right-hand entry to the next right-hand entry).
- *Stroke rate* (or stroke frequency): The number of stroke cycles per minute.
- *Swimming speed* (or velocity)
- *Split times* (each 25/50 m segment of the race)

Interpretation

Interpretation of physiological testing with individual swimmers should account for a wide range of factors that can influence results. The most obvious of these factors are age (chronological age), gender (male or female), and characteristics of the underlying event including distance (sprint, middle-distance, or distance) and stroke (freestyle, form stroke, or individual medley). The immediate (previous weeks to months) and long-term (years of training and competitive experience) training history of the swimmer should also be considered. Testing during the competitive and championships seasons is likely to see the swimmer in a

Table 8.5 Benchmarking of 100- and 200-m freestyle (long course) world records for men's and women's events showing 50-m split times, cumulative time, and final race time.

Event	Men		Women	
	Cumulative time	Final race time	Cumulative time	Final race time
100-m Freestyle				
Name	Pieter van den Hoogenband (NED)		Libby Lenton (AUS)	
Date	19 Sept 2000		31 March 2004	
50 m	23.16	23.16	25.81	25.81
100 m	47.84	24.68	53.66	27.85
200-m Backstroke				
Name	Aaron Piersol (USA)		Kristina Egerszegi (HUN)	
Date	20 March 2002		25 Aug 1991	
50 m	27.75	27.75	30.55	30.55
100 m	56.60	28.85	1.02.34	31.79
150 m	1.26.05	29.45	1.34.79	32.45
200 m	1.55.15	29.10	2.06.62	31.83

different physiological condition compared with the pre-season or early season when the swimmer is coming off a break. The coach and swimmer should have some expectation whether tests results are likely to show improvement, maintenance, or degradation in the level of fitness. In general, swimmers should be able to swim within 4–5% of their expected race time in training throughout the season. This equates to approximately 2–3 s for 100-m events, 4–5 s for 200-m events, and 10–12 s for 400-m events. The presence of any underlying or preexisting illness, injury, or fatigue should be noted and considered.

A major limitation of testing is where physiological results are interpreted in isolation, rather than considering performance and physiological responses in parallel. For example, the results of heart rate and lactate responses are often interpreted without consideration of the underlying characteristics of performance (i.e., total times, split times, percentage of personal best time) and stroke efficiency (i.e., fluctuations in stroke rate and stroke count). A measurable change in heart rate or blood lactate concentration may well reflect variability in technique (from the interaction of propulsive power and drag forces) rather than a change

Table 8.6 Competition analysis for the first three swimmers in the final of the men's and women's 100-m freestyle at the 1998 FINA World Swimming Championships. Race components include stroke length, stroke frequency (number of stroke cycles per minute), start time (first 15 m), turn time (7.5 m in and out of the turn), time for the final 25 m, and finish time (last 5 m).

Race component	Men's 100-m freestyle			Women's 100-m freestyle		
	Alex Popov	Michael Klim	Lars Frolander	Jenny Thompson	Martina Moravcova	Ying Shan
Stroke length						
1st 25	2.49 m	2.31 m	2.34 m	2.09 m	1.73 m	1.87 m
2nd 25	2.57 m	2.37 m	2.14 m	1.97 m	1.94 m	1.96 m
3rd 25	2.6 m	2.29 m	2.14 m	1.89 m	1.98 m	2.0 m
4th 25	2.29 m	2.26 m	2.0 m	1.9 m	1.89 m	2.0 m
Average for race	2.49 m	2.31 m	2.16 m	1.96 m	1.89 m	1.96 m
Stroke frequency (strokes · min^{-1})	48.8	51.2	54.3	52.2	53.4	53.0
Start time (15 m)	5.86 s	6.08 s	6.26 s	6.75 s	7.05 s	6.71 s
Turn time (15 m)	7.12 s	7.08 s	7.12 s	7.80 s	8.08 s	8.04 s
Last 25 m time	13.31 s	13.22 s	13.23 s	14.45 s	13.55 s	13.82 s
Finish time (5 m)	2.49 s	2.48 s	2.29 s	2.62 s	2.96 s	2.59 s

in underlying fitness characteristics *per se*. It is essential that the results of physiological testing are interpreted in light of the relevant performance and stroke mechanics data.

Future directions

The physiological testing of elite swimmers has evolved greatly over the last half century, and at the start of the new millennium it appears that the rate of progress will be maintained. The 1960s and 1970s was the era of whole body physiological and cardiorespiratory testing of athletes (Baldwin 2000). In swimming this was characterized by measurement of parameters such as heart rate, lung function, body temperature, and aerobic capacity. The 1980s and 1990s was seen as the era of cellular biochemistry with emphasis on hematological and biochemical testing. The most visible manifestation of this era was the introduction of blood lactate testing in the preparation of highly trained swimmers (Madsen & Lohberg 1987). At the dawn of the twenty-first century, genetic modeling of physiological factors that affect sport performance is a very active field of scientific endeavor. A number of genes have already been identified that identify the genetic predisposition of athletes for endurance (angiotensin converting enzyme (Myerson 1999)) and sprint (α-actinin3 (North 1999)) activities. Despite the rapid pace of developments in science, medicine, and technology, the testing of swimmers will continue to reflect a balance between research outcomes and the hard-earned practical experience of swimmers and coaches.

References

Baldwin, K.M. (2000) Research in the exercise sciences: where do we go from here? *Journal of Applied Physiology* **88**, 332–336.

Bishop, D., Jenkins, D.G. & Mackinnon, L.T. (1998) The relationship between plasma lactate parameters, Wpeak and 1-h cycling performance in women. *Medicine and Science in Sports and Exercise* **30**, 1270–1275.

Counsilman, B.E. & Counsilman, J.E. (1991) The residual effects of training. *Journal of Swimming Research* **7**, 5–12.

Counsilman, B.E. & Counsilman, J.E. (1993) Problems

with the physiological classification of endurance loads. *American Swimming Magazine* Dec/Jan, 4–20.

Foster, C. (1998) Monitoring training in athletes with reference to the overtraining syndrome. *Medicine and Science in Sports and Exercise* **30**, 1164–1168.

Hawes, M.R. & Sovak, D. (1994) Morphological prototypes, assessment and change in elite athletes. *Journal of Sports Science* **12**, 234–242.

Hopkins, W.G., Hawley, J.A. & Burke, L.M. (1999) Design and analysis of research on sport performance enhancement. *Medicine and Science in Sports and Exercise* **31**, 472–485.

Madsen, O. & Lohberg, M. (1987) The lowdown on lactates. *Swimming Technique* May–July, 21–25.

Mason, B.R. (1999) Biomechanical race analysis. In: *31st American Swimming Coaches Association Annual World Clinic*, San Diego, California, pp. 99–114.

Meleski, B.W. & Malina, R.M. (1985) Changes in body composition and physique of elite university-level female swimmers during a competitive season. *Journal of Sports Science* **3**, 33–40.

Mujika, I. & Padilla, S. (2000) Detraining: loss of training-induced physiological and performance adaptations. Part 1. *Sports Medicine* **30**, 79–87.

Mujika, I., Busso, T., Lacoste, L., Barale, F., Geyssant, A. & Chatard, J.-C. (1996) Modelled responses to training and taper in competitive swimmers. *Medicine and Science in Sports and Exercise* **28**, 251–258.

Mujika, I., Padilla, S. & Pyne, D. (2002) Swimming performance changes during the final 3 weeks of training leading to the Sydney 2000 Olympic Games. *International Journal of Sports Medicine* **23**(8), 582–587.

Myerson, S., Hemingway, H., Budget, R., Martin, J., Humphries, S. & Montgomery, H. (1999) Human angiotensin I-converting enzyme gene and endurance performance. *Journal of Applied Physiology* **87**, 1313–1316.

North, K. (1999) Genetic influences on athletic performance. In: *5th IOC World Congress on Sport Sciences*, Sydney, Australia. (Abstract.)

Prins, J. (1988) Setting a standard. *Swimming Technique* May–July, 13–17.

Pyne, D.B., Maw, G.J. & Goldsmith, W.M. (2000) Protocols for the physiological assessment of swimmers. In: C.J. Gore, ed. *Protocols for the Physiological assessment of Swimmers*. Champaign, IL: Human Kinetics, pp. 372–382.

Pyne, D.B., Trewin, C.B. & Hopkins, W.G. (in press) Progression and variability in competitive performance of Olympic swimmers. *Journal of Sports Sciences*.

Sleivert, G. & Mackinnon, L.T. (1991) The validation of backward extrapolation of submaximal oxygen consumption from the oxygen recovery curve. *European Journal of Applied Physiology* **63**, 135–139.

Snyder, A.C., Jeukendrup, A.E., Hesselink, M.K.C., Kuipers, H. & Foster, C. (1993) A physiological/psychological indicator of over-reaching during intensive training. *International Journal of Sports Medicine* **14**, 29–32.

Stewart, A.M. & Hopkins, W.G. (2000) Consistency of swimming performance within and between competitions. *Medicine and Science in Sports and Exercise* **32**(5), 997–1001.

Trappe, S., Costill, D. & Thomas, R. (2000) Effect of swim taper on whole muscle and single muscle fiber contractile properties. *Medicine and Science in Sports and Exercise* **32**, 48–56.

Trewin, C., Pyne, D.B. & Hopkins, W. (2004) Relationship between world-ranking and Olympic performance of swimmers in the 2000 Olympic Games. *Journal of Sports Sciences* **22**, 339–345.

Troup, J.P. (1999) The physiology and biomechanics of competitive swimming. *Aquatic Sports Injuries and Rehabilitation*. **18**, 267–285.

Weltman, A. (1993) *The Blood Lactate Response to Exercise*. Champaign, IL: Human Kinetics, pp. 85–92.

Index

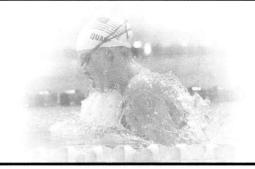